A CENTURY OF
PORTUGUESE FERTILITY

This book is the first in a projected series on
the decline of European fertility.
A Publication of the Office of Population Research
Princeton University

A Century of Portuguese Fertility

BY MASSIMO LIVI BACCI

PRINCETON UNIVERSITY PRESS
PRINCETON, N.J. 1971

LCC 70-120758
ISBN 978-0-691-64734-0

Publication of this book has been aided
by the Whitney Darrow Publication Reserve Fund of
Princeton University Press

This book has been composed in Linotype Times Roman

Printed in the United States of America
by Princeton University Press

Foreword

In 1964 the Office of Population Research at Princeton embarked on an extended study of the modern decline of fertility in Europe. The project originated in the realization that every country in Europe, and indeed almost every one of the more than 700 provinces in Europe, has very substantially lower birth rates than in the fairly recent past. In most provinces, in fact, the number of children born per woman is no more than half what it was a century or so ago. This pervasive change is an important part of the social history of Europe because a major change in fertility necessarily implies a different role for women, a reorganization of families, a profoundly different age structure of the population, and changes in many other characteristics of society.

The decline of fertility has special interest for demographers because one of the best known generalizations in demography is that modernization and industrialization tend to be accompanied by a drastic decrease in the rate of childbearing. The several hundred provinces of Europe can be viewed as a statistical laboratory in which hypotheses about the social and economic circumstances under which fertility declines can be tested. European statistics of population are unusually complete and accurate, although far from perfect, and the decline in fertility has occurred under widely different circumstances and at dates that range from before 1800 to after World War II.

The organization of the project calls for separate studies of individual countries or regions and for a final examination of the experience in Europe as a whole. It was the good fortune of the Office of Population Research that Professor Massimo Livi Bacci of the University of Florence agreed to study the fall of fertility in Italy, Spain, and Portugal. This book on Portugal, then, is the first of a series of country studies in which we plan future publications on France, Germany, Austria, Hungary and the Balkans, and Russia. The final book of the series will be a synthesis for all of Europe.

FOREWORD

In his study of Portugal the author has found strong contrasts in age at marriage, the proportion remaining single, and marital fertility in the different provinces, and also has found substantial differences in the time at which marital fertility began to decline. Conventional explanations of declining fertility, invoking the effects of increasing education and changing occupational structure, for example, are at best weakly confirmed. Professor Livi Bacci has given us a clear picture of recent demographic changes in Portugal, but properly attempts only a partial causal explanation, and ends with tentative and speculative conclusions.

Ansley J. Coale
Director
Office of Population Research

Contents

List of Tables

List of Figures

A CENTURY OF PORTUGUESE FERTILITY

CHAPTER 1: Environment and Society: An Introductory Outline

1.1. *General Traits of Portugal*

In western Europe, Portugal is probably the country least known and studied by social scientists, although it represents a very interesting case study in view of its peculiar development. Our study aims to cover an important part of the social and demographic history of the country, and is mainly concerned with the transition from a situation of high, almost uncontrolled fertility to the moderate pattern prevailing in recent times. In addition, we offer an analysis of the peculiarities and changes of Portuguese society that have determined, directly or indirectly, the decline of fertility.

This introductory chapter therefore outlines the environmental conditions of the society where this transition from high to moderate fertility has taken place, including the geographical setting, the distribution and forms of exploitation of the land, the system of communication, and regional uniformities and contrasts. It is obvious that each one of these topics could be the subject of a separate study, but our aim is merely to provide the reader with the background information necessary for an understanding of fertility trends and differentials.

Portugal is still a very backward country, at least in comparison with the other countries of Western civilization and in spite of the improvements of the last decades. Its per capita income is the lowest in western Europe. Illiteracy, infant mortality, and the incidence of infectious diseases are at the highest level. Only in some areas of the Balkans (Albania, Southern Yugoslavia) do conditions similar to those of Portugal still exist. These conditions in the Balkans derive, however, from centuries of isolation under Turkish rule, and are not the heritage—as in Portugal—of the decline of a great political power.

Portugal is an isolated society; its geographical position at the southwestern end of Europe, the slow diffusion of mass communication media, the political barriers set up by its authoritarian governments against free cultural contacts and exchanges with the outer world, have deeply affected the development of the country, even preserving, in certain areas, features and customs of an archaic, premodern society. The isolation of the country from the rest of Europe became more evident when, with the end of colonial expansion, the balance of political and economic power of the continent shifted to the north. Portugal was then further away from the mainstream of Western thought, culture, and fashions. Even contacts with Spain have always been weak, more because of historical events than because of geographical barriers. Moreover, the least developed areas in Spain are those that border on Portugal.

Many demographers view the process of transition from high to low fertility as the result of a diffusion of a new psychological attitude towards procreation, fostered by social and territorial mobility and by the often complex and tight contacts between countries. It is probably correct to say that in Portugal the development of a pattern of moderate fertility has taken place in an autonomous way, owing little or nothing to external influence. It is true that Portuguese society shared many of the features of the south European, Mediterranean culture, but its isolation from the rest of Europe makes the hypothesis very plausible that fertility control has developed following an endogenous process, relatively free from outside influence. This may be an advantage to us, because one of the complicating factors often encountered in interpreting the decline of fertility can be eliminated from the start.

1.2. *Geographical Outline*

Some indication, if only in summary form, of the geographical characteristics of Portugal are a necessary introduction to the demographic study that we intend to undertake.[1] A country of almost rectangular shape, accounting for about 15 percent of the entire

[1] For a comprehensive outline of Portuguese geography, see O. Ribeiro, "Portugal," in *Geografía de España y Portugal*, edited by M. de Teran, Vol. v, Barcelona, 1955. See also P. Birot, *Le Portugal. Etude de géographie régionale*, Paris, 1950; A. Blanc, M. Drain, B. Kayser, *L'Europe Méditerranéenne*, Paris, 1967; J. Vilá Valenti, *La Péninsule Ibérique*, Paris, 1968.

Iberian peninsula, it is predominantly mountainous in the northeastern section, where the Meseta extends towards the coast and forms a series of fanshaped mountain chains which stretch from Galicia in a southwesterly direction. Although the mountain chains are not very high, the terrain is very rough, and forms a substantial obstacle to longitudinal communications. The area marked by the influence of the mountains extends to the valleys of the Zézere and the Tagus rivers, and includes the provinces of Tras-os-Montes/Alto Douro and the Beira Alta, but excludes the Minho, and the littorals of the Douro and Beira, forming a longitudinal coastal plain bordering the ocean. Plains and low plateaus are predominant in the south, which includes the whole area below the Tagus, the valley of this river (Ribatejo) and Estremadura. South of the Tagus stretches the low plateau of the Alentejo, which is separated from the southern coast—the Algarve—by a series of hills forming an amphitheatre facing the sea.

The country is also deeply influenced by the rivers which cross it and which, in part, form its borders. To the north, the Minho forms in its final course the border between Spain and Portugal; to the east, the Douro, Tagus, and Guadiana outline part of the border. The Douro and the Tagus have for centuries set the boundaries between the major regional areas of the country (north of the Douro: regions of Minho and Tras-os-Montes; between the Douro and the Tagus: regions of Beira and Estremadura; south of the Tagus: regions of Alentejo and Algarve), a distinction discarded by modern geographers,[2] but historically based on the successive waves of the reconquest of the country from Moorish domination. The Minho, Lima, Douro, Mondego, and Tagus cross the country with a southwesterly orientation; all rivers north of the Tagus flow through deep valleys and gorges, making communications between north and south rather difficult. They become navigable towards their mouths, thus forming waterways favorable to communication and transportation.

The regional structure of Portugal, however, is determined not only by the nature of the relief and waterways but also by the

[2] A. de Amorim Girão, *Geografia de Portugal*, Porto, 1941.

varying characteristics of the climate. According to Ribeiro,[3] an imaginary line separates the north from the south, following the course of the Mondego from the sea to Coimbra, then forming an ample circle bordering the southern edge of the central mountain chain and reaching the Spanish border north of Penamacor. South of this imaginary line, the unifying action of the Mediterranean influence renders the climatic characteristics of the area homogeneous, marked by the scarcity of rain and a long, hot, dry summer. The north is less homogeneous from a climatic point of view. The northeastern, mountainous section (Tras-os-Montes, Alto Douro, and Beira Alta) is essentially subjected to a continental climate, while the northwestern part of the area is subjected to the moderate Atlantic weather system, and has abundant rainfall. In the north of the country a vegetation of the Atlantic type prevails and forests are frequent; the method of soil cultivation is ancient and the distribution of land very fragmented; abundant rainfall and irrigation facilities produce a system of diverse crops; and, the population is sparsely settled.[4] These characteristics cannot be found in the south (with the exception of Estremadura and Algarve), where the distribution of the land is concentrated, the agriculture is predominantly monocultural (cereals, olives), the cultivation of the soil is relatively recent, and the population is clustered in large rural villages.

The relationships between the geographical characteristics and the demographic development of the different regions cannot be shown here; but the reader will note that basic geographic differences exist, that they have deeply affected the rural economy and the rural life of the various regions and have therefore to be taken into account when studying social and demographic changes.

1.3. *Geographical and Administrative Subdivisions*

Until the beginning of the nineteenth century, historians and geographers subdivided Portugal into six regions: Minho, Tras-os-Montes, Beira, Estremadura, Alentejo, and Algarve. The geographic limits of the six regions have always been uncertain and

[3] Ribeiro, *op. cit.*, p. 235.

[4] Vilá Valenti, *op. cit.*, p. 242.

have varied through time, since they did not have any political, administrative, or legal significance.[5] At the beginning of the last century, the six regions were subdivided into forty-four *comarcas* having some administrative functions.[6]

In 1836, the liberal regime introduced a new administrative unit, the *distrito*, grouping several *concelhos* with characteristics and prerogatives similar to the Spanish municipalities and to the Italian communes; each *concelho* is formed by one or more *freguezias* (parishes). The subdivision into districts—seventeen on the continent and four in the islands (three for the Azores and one for Madeira)—has remained virtually unchanged until now, with the exception of the introduction of the district of Setúbal, in 1926, by separation from Lisbon (see Fig. 1). This constancy facilitates the study that we intend to undertake and assures the possibility of comparisons through time. The administrative subdivision of the country was challenged and discussed several times, and projects of reformation were often advanced (in 1842, 1867, and 1914, for instance) but never actuated.[7] In fact, the *distritos*, created for administrative purposes, often do not have homogeneous geographic and environmental characteristics; in this regard they have been the object of criticism by geographers and social scientists.[8] However, the administrative and economic functions which are concentrated (since 1836) in the capital of the districts have succeeded, in their own way, in influencing the development of the surrounding territory; therefore, a redistribution of the population into geographically similar areas, according to other criteria, would not be justified.

In 1936, the new civil code superimposed on the existing districts eleven *provincias*; since there is no correspondence between the confines of the two types of administrative areas, there are

[5] A. Balbi, *Compendio di geografía*, Vol. I, Turin, 1840.

[6] For a history of the geographical, political, and administrative subdivision of Portugal, see E. de Castro Caldas and M. de Santos Loureiro, *Regioes homogéneas no continente Português*, Lisbon, 1966.

[7] *Ibid.*, pp. 89-95.

[8] G. Ferro, "Le frontiere del Portogallo e la sua suddivisione regionale," in *Rivista geografica Italiana*, Vol. LXXI (1964), pp. 113-114.

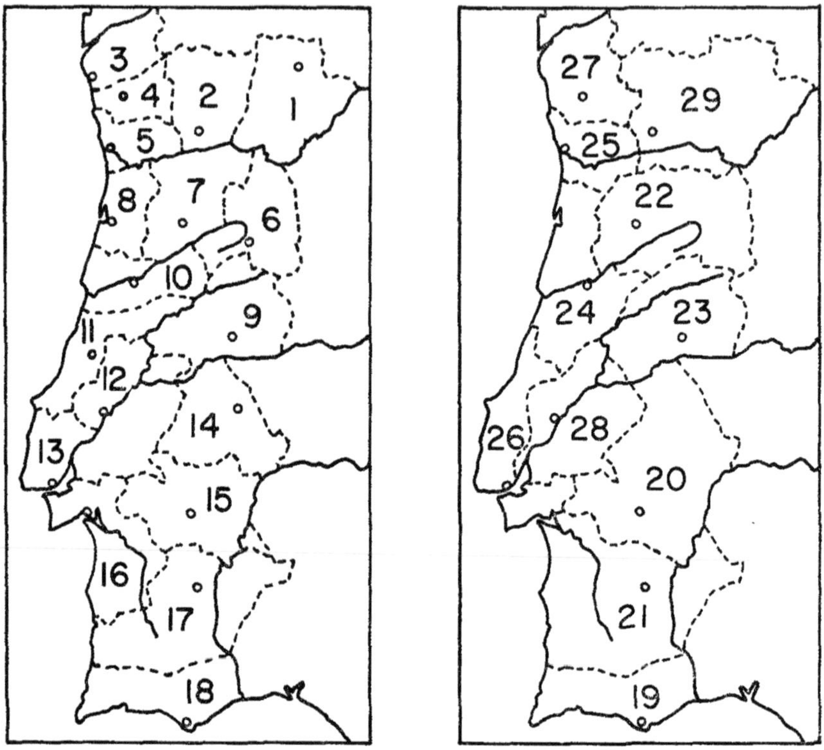

Figure 1. Administrative subdivisions of Portugal: districts and provinces

A—continental districts

1. Bragança
2. Vila Real
3. Viana do Castelo
4. Braga
5. Porto
6. Guarda
7. Viseu
8. Aveiro
9. Castelo Branco
10. Coimbra
11. Leiria
12. Santarém
13. Lisbon
14. Portalegre
15. Évora
16. Setúbal
17. Beja
18. Faro

B—continental provinces

19. Algarve
20. Alto Alentejo
21. Baixo Alentejo
22. Beira Alta
23. Beira Baixa
24. Beira Litoral
25. Douro Litoral
26. Estremadura
27. Minho
28. Ribatejo
29. Tras-os-Montes e Alto Douro

districts belonging to different provinces. The creation of the provinces derives from the work of the geographer Amorim Girão; in his conception the rivers are considered as unifying factors of the economic and social life of the different regions and not as elements of separation.[9] Other geographers (Lautensach, Albuquerque, Ribeiro) have proposed different criteria of regionalization. Because we thought it of special interest, we presented in the preceding section Ribeiro's idea, which stresses the basic differences existing between the north Transmontano and the Atlantic on one side, and the south Mediterranean on the other.

1.4. *Communications and Mobility*

We have said at the beginning that isolation is one of the distinctive marks of the Portuguese society. Even contacts with Spain have always been rare, although there are no important geographical barriers between the two countries, at least not along the extensive eastern border. But unfortunately for Portugal, the regions bordering on Portugal are themselves the least developed in Spain; Galicia to the north; Leon, Spanish Estremadura, and western Andalusia to the east. On both sides of the border the population density is very low; contact between the two countries has consisted solely of permanent migration of Galicians to the Portuguese towns, and seasonal migration from Algarve to Andalusia for summer crops. Contacts with the rest of the world were, during most of the nineteenth century, limited to sea traffic; it was only in 1876 that Lisbon was connected with the rest of Europe by rail, via Salamanca.[10]

The situation of internal communications at mid-nineteenth century was equally poor. Pery observes that the only good road in 1851 was the short Lisbon-Sintra stretch, connecting two royal residences.[11] Regular communications between the two major cities, Lisbon and Porto, were possible only by boat; the trip by land took several days of uncomfortable traveling on horseback or stagecoach

[9] Castro Caldas and Santos Loureiro, *op. cit.*, p. 97.
[10] Ribeiro, *op. cit.*, p. 204.
[11] Aranha and others, *Le Portugal*, Paris, no date, p. 121.

on ill-kept roads and remnants of Roman highways.[12] It was only in 1864 that Lisbon was connected with Porto by railroad; the construction of the network proceeded slowly at the beginning (only 967 km. in 1875), then with an accelerated pace; by the beginning of the First World War 3,135 km. of the current total of 3,589 had been completed.

The whole social and economic life of the country has centered during the last century on the Lisbon-Porto axis and the surrounding area, between the Tagus and the Douro, a region equipped with an efficient system of communications and receiving the strong stimuli of the two largest cities of the country. Ribeiro views the dynamism of Portugal as concentrated in the coastal strip between Lisbon and Porto, extended northward to Braga and southward to Setúbal, and penetrating the inner country along the valleys of the Tagus, Mondego, and Douro.[13] The other dynamic area of the country, the southern Algarvian litoral, is virtually autonomous from the rest of the country. It is interesting to note that the Algarve was almost completely isolated until the completion of the railway connecting Lisbon with Faro in 1889. Before this date, contacts with the rest of the country were possible only by sea, and until 1875 only by sailboats. The first motor road connecting Faro with Beja came much later, being finished only in 1922.[14]

At the other end of the country, the northeastern Tras-os-Montes was equally isolated from the rest of the country, especially because of the mountainous nature of the region. Until the end of the nineteenth century the region was not part of the railway network, and two of the three lines serving the main valleys of the Tras-os-Montes —the valley of the Corgo line and the Mogadouro line—were completed in 1922 and 1930.[15]

The railroad network could serve the basic needs of the country by the beginning of the First World War, but roads were rare and

[12] Ribeiro, *op. cit.*, p. 204. [13] *Ibid.*, pp. 204-205.

[14] M. Feio, "Le bas Alentejo et l'Algarve," *Congrès international de géographie*, Lisbon, 1949, p. 148.

[15] Blanc, Drain and Kayser, *op. cit.*, p. 74.

in very poor condition. It is only in the last three decades that a conspicuous effort has been made to create an efficient system of highways.

It is obvious that the slow progress of the communications system, the difficulty of contacts of the peripheral regions with the rest of the country until relatively recent times, together with the natural obstacles set by rivers and mountains, are all factors in the slow social development of certain areas of the country, in the preservation of their ethnic and cultural peculiarities, and also in the prevention of the development of internal mobility. We will see in due course that these facts are not irrelevant to the history of regional fertility.

1.5. *Elements of Regional Differentiation*

It has been observed already that the regional geographical and climatic differences have produced substantial disparities as far as the régime of land distribution is concerned.[16] There is no doubt that the plains of the south are more fit for extensive cultivation in large economic units than the mountains and valleys prevailing in the northeast of the country. Moreover, the reconquest of the south from the Moorish domination was followed by the distribution of land to the Church, the military orders, and the aristocracy, causing a strong concentration of land in the hands of a few owners, a situation surviving until today in spite of the selling of the Church and military properties in the nineteenth century. On the other hand, in the Minho, the ancient occupation of the soil, the abundant rainfall, and the irrigation facilities—which make possible an intensive and diverse cultivation of the land—have resulted in the increasing fragmentation of the properties. In Tras-os-Montes and Beira there still survive types of communal ownership and exploitation of land and pastures, once characteristic of the whole area and deeply influencing many aspects of the *transmontana* society.

The average dimension of the farm unit is only 2.1 ha. in the

[16] *Ibid.*, p. 74.

north, 3.5 in the center, 39.6 in the south (excluding the Algarve), and 5.3 in Algarve.[17] In the north, and particularly in the Minho, the farm workers are in the great majority also farmholders. The property is generally entailed in equal shares to the sons, thus producing an ever-increasing fragmentation of land. The small size of the holdings produces a continuous emigration, particularly of males. The women are frequently employed in agriculture, not only as a consequence of the emigration of males, but also because the diversified type of cultivation requires the year-round care of all members of the family.[18] In the south, and particularly in the Alentejo, the great majority of the labor force consists of hired laborers, often living on the farm while the wife and children remain in the village. The women generally attend to housework and are seldom engaged in other activities.[19]

There are basic differences in the psychology of the inhabitants of the Minho and of the Alentejo other than those related to the organization of agriculture.[20] Loyalty to tradition and religion is a distinctive characteristic of the people of the Minho, where the city of Braga is considered the religious center of the country; religious vocations are more frequent than in other areas, and folklore is rich in religious elements. Family ties are very strong in spite of frequent separations of husband and wife due to migration, and the Minhoto is generally described as conservative and suspicious toward any kind of innovation—traits commonly ascribed to populations where proprietors, no matter how poor and miserable they are, are numerically very important.[21] The character of the Alentejano is very different. The social class of proprietors and tenants, because of the prevalence of latifundia, is numerically negligible. Family ties are less extended and strong; the hold of the Church

[17] O.C.D.E., "Le Portugal," in *Études économiques de l'O.C.D.E.*, Paris, 1964, Table IV, p. 28.

[18] J. Dias, "Minho, Tras-os-Montes, Haut Douro," *Congrès international de géographie*, Lisbon, 1949, pp. 18, 118-120.

[19] Feio, *op. cit.*, passim.

[20] For a description of the psychological traits of the regional populations see P. Descamps, *Le Portugal*, Paris, 1935, pp. 64-232. See also, F. Villier, *Portogallo*, Milan, 1961.

[21] Descamps, *op. cit.*, pp. 85-89.

on the population is neither firm nor tight. Frequently, couples get married with only civil rites; sometimes they do not even bother to get married. Church attendance is low, atheism frequent.[22] Poinsard and Descamps have pointed out the unstable character of the family in the Alentejo, as opposed to the stability of the family in the Minho.

THE VERY summary notes presented here describe the existence of two different poles of Portuguese society: the Minho and the Alentejo, two regions that with a further simplification can be assumed to represent the characteristics of the north and of the south, although there is a large area of transition in between where identification with one or the other of the two types is impossible because of the mobility of the population and the dynamism of the society. Still, in the hearts of the north and of the south are evident variations of the model described above. In the northeast, where long isolation has preserved many of its distinctive characteristics, the tradition of a communal social and economic life has certainly strengthened family ties and deepened attachment to the clan. At the very south of the country, the Algarvian society is, in many aspects, different from the Alentejano type. The property is more fragmented and latifundia more rare; there is a large class of farm owners and tenants, and the prosperity of the activities related to fishing constitutes another distinctive mark of the area. The society still bears the marks of Moorish domination and has evolved independent of external influences, in part because of its physical isolation. In spite of such differences, family ties are not very tight, and religiosity is low—as in Alentejo.

The reader must be aware of the simplifications we have introduced into this chapter in an effort to give a short account of the basic characteristics of the country, of the regional similarities and contrasts. In due course we will come back, in more detail, to some of the topics delineated in these pages.

[22] *Ibid.*, pp. 192-193, 213.

Chapter 2: Population Development During the Nineteenth Century

2.1. *Population Growth During the Nineteenth Century*

Information on the Portuguese population before 1864, year of the first modern census, is not abundant.[1] The cadastral enumeration of 1527, during the reign of João III, is the earliest source of a reliable estimate of the population of the country. At that time around 290,000 households were enumerated, but the lack of precise information as to the size of the household makes it very difficult to convert this figure into total population. However, we would not be too far from the truth estimating a total population of around 1.2 million. The later enumerations of 1636 and, under the Spanish rule, of 1732, have been considered by most scholars to be scanty and unreliable. By 1768 another enumeration whose exact nature is still debated put the total number of households at 633,000 and the total population around 2.4 million, about double the approximation of 150 years before. The enumeration of Pina Manique (1798) again gave only the total number of households (746,864).

In 1801 the census promoted by the Count of Linhares gives a fairly detailed analysis of the number of households and the population, by sex, for every administrative unit.[2] After that date there

[1] For a history of the population of Portugal, see especially Soares de Barros, "Sobre a causa da diferente população em diversos tempos da Monarchia," in *Memorias economicas da Academia Real das Sciências de Lisboa*, Vol. I, 1789, pp. 123-151. The best critical study is by the Italian geographer A. Balbi, *Essai statistique sur le royaume de Portugal et d'Algarve, comparé aux autres états de l'Europe, et suivi d'un coup d'oeil sur l'état actuel des sciences, des lettres et des beaux arts parmi les Portugais des deux hémisphères*, Paris, 1822, Vol. I, pp. 184-241. See also, by the same author, *Variétés politico-statistiques sur la monarchie Portugaise*, Paris, 1822.

For a summary of the historical material on population, Estatística de Portugal, População, *Censo no 1° de janeiro de 1864*, Lisbon, 1868, p. xvi; Instituto Nacional de Estatística, *VIII recenseamento geral da população no continente e ilhas adjacentes em 12 de dezembro 1940*, Vol. XXIV-XXV, Lisbon, 1945, pp. 19-21. A critical appraisal of the statistical sources on population in the eighteenth and early nineteenth centuries, may be found in A. Silbert, *Le Portugal Méditerranéen*, Vol. I, S.E.V.P.E.N., Paris, 1966, pp. 105-120.

[2] Instituto Nacional de Estatística, *Subsídios para a história da estatística em*

are several enumerations (1821, 1835, 1838, 1841, 1854, 1858. 1861) of the Portuguese population, mostly of an administrative or fiscal nature, before the 1864 census, the first with modern characteristics. The enumeration of 1864 was nominative and individual; it was taken simultaneously throughout the national territory and followed by other censuses in 1878, 1890, and 1900.

In Table 1[3] we have reported the number of households and the population from 1768 to 1900, and the corresponding growth rates.

Table 1. Population and Households in Continental Portugal, 1768-1900

Year	Households (000)	Population (000)	Rate of growth: (percent) Households	Population
1768	633.4	--	--	--
1801	758.5	2,931	.55	--
1820	765.4	3,013	.05	.15
1841	840.9	3,397	.45	.55
1864	958.2	3,830	.57	.52
1878	1,040.6	4,160	.61	.62
1890	1,151.6	4,660	.89	1.00
1900	1,205.8	5,016	.47	.76

On the whole, an accelerated growth can be observed throughout the period; the slow development during the first two decades of the nineteenth century is probably the consequence of the wars fought then in connection with the French invasion.[4] The acceleration during the second half of the century—although the effects of an increasing completeness of the enumeration cannot be excluded

Portugal, Vol. II, *Taboas topograficas e estatísticas 1801*, Lisbon, 1948. It is the edition of the manuscript edited by Manuel Travassos, and based on the results of the enumeration ordered by the Count of Linhares.

[3] The data are drawn from Instituto Nacional de Estatística, *Anuário demográfico 1950*, Lisbon, 1951, p. 6.

[4] See Silbert, *op. cit.*, p. 117; and Balbi, "Essai," *op. cit.*, Vol. I, pp. 193ff.

—is probably to be imputed to declining mortality, since the birth rate, as we will see in the following paragraph, had remained almost stable during the century. An average rate of growth slightly above .5 percent over the nineteenth century is well in line with the type of growth prevailing during the same period in the Mediterranean countries.

2.2 *Births and Birth Rates at the Beginning of the Nineteenth Century*

Although the first "modern" census dates back to 1864, statistics of demographic events such as births, deaths, and marriages started being compiled on a continuing basis only at the end of the century (1886). During the century, however, some statistics of vital events were produced occasionally from either official or unofficial sources. Their quality, reliability, and territorial disaggregation is extremely variable, but they offer precious information which has to be taken into account and carefully evaluated.

The first source is the enumeration of the population and the households of 1801, carried out in 1802, and based on lists provided by civil and religious authorities. Besides the data on population and households, the enumeration includes data on births and deaths in the year 1801. The Instituto Nacional de Estatística published in 1948 a copy of the manuscript containing the results of the enumeration, compiled by Manuel Travassos, and containing also a recapitulation of vital events for the forty-four *comarcas*, subdivisions of the six provinces.[5] Balbi reports, in his basic work on Portugal, the same data and other data referring to the same year but compiled by ecclesiastical subdivisions.[6] These last figures do not coincide with those produced by Travassos, as can be seen below:

Author	*Households*	*Population*	*Births*	*Deaths*
Travassos	758,501	2,931,393	95,407	90,071
Balbi (ecclesiastical subdivision)	749,524	2,875,413	97,539	89,567

[5] See note 2. The recapitulation for the 44 *comarcas* is presented in the final table, "Estado da Povoação de Portugal no anno de 1801 para 1802."

[6] Balbi, "Essai," *op. cit.*, pp. 204-205.

The lower figures given by Balbi are justified because of the omission from the count of the parishes under the jurisdiction of the "dignitaires exempts."[7] However, Balbi's higher figure for births is surprising, and probably imputable to a more careful collection of the parish records kept by the religious authorities.

The data for 1801 may be supplemented with the data collected under the direction of Colonel Franzini in 1822, concerning the population of the administrative units in 1819, and the number of households, births, deaths, and marriages for the 1815-1819 period. The only trace of these data is provided by Balbi,[8] but for only twenty-four of the forty-four *comarcas*, covering about 53 percent of the total population (from a minimum of 36 percent for Beira to a maximum of 100 percent for Algarve). It is possible, therefore, to compute the birth rates for the 6 provinces in 1801 and 1815-1819. For 1801 we give the values based either on Travassos' or Balbi's data. The data reported in Table 2, however, are not comparable for the following reasons:

(1) The two evaluations for 1801—civil and ecclesiastical—refer to noncoincident subdivisions of the country.
(2) The comparison between Travassos' data for 1801 and the 1815-1819 figures, although geographically correct, is affected by the incomplete coverage of the 1815-1819 data.

The quality of the data is difficult to evaluate. Balbi himself had some doubts as to their precision and reliability. He warns that from the number of registered births (baptisms) was excluded a fraction of infants who died shortly after birth.[9] On the other hand, the number of foundlings included at least 5 percent of the cases of infants already baptized;[10] this proportion of births, if added to the statistics of the baptized, would have caused a slight duplication.

[7] Santa Cruz de Douro, Royal Chapel of Vila Vicosa, the Monasteries of San João de Taruoca, San Cristovão de Lafôès, and San Pedro de Aguias (at least 24 parishes) were "exempted" and excluded from the count. The enumeration is defective for the "exempted" areas of Crato: Thomar, Santa Cruz de Coimbra and Grijo. See Balbi, "Essai," *op. cit.*, p. 206.

[8] *Ibid.*, pp. 192-93, 207-210.

[9] *Ibid.*, p. 211.

[10] *Ibid.*, p. 212.

The enumerations of deaths were, according to Balbi, much more incomplete, since the priests "do not always take note of the deaths of the children of the poor, dead before the age of communion, whose corpses are deposited at the doors of the churches by the parents who want to avoid the expenses of the burial," not to speak of the deaths in the monasteries, excluded from the count. Balbi concludes that "these facts, together with the great ignorance of some priests, and with the natural dislike that each priest has for any enumeration of inhabitants and for any kind of calculations, mean that the Portuguese lists (of vital events) are very inexact, and offer only very approximate data, especially as far as the deaths in the large cities are concerned."[11] We have extensively quoted Balbi's opinions about Portuguese statistics because they are probably true, especially for death statistics, until the end of the century.

Table 2 contains data on population, households, birth rates, and the sex ratio at birth for the six provinces in 1801 and from 1815 to 1819. Balbi himself warns against the superficial interpretation of the 1801 data: "a bad year (1801) because of the famine which desolated the country and which certainly powerfully influenced the growth of the population."[12] Both in 1801 and 1815-1819, the birth rate was much higher in the south (Alentejo, Algarve) than in the north of the country. It is, however, uncertain, whether the differences in the birth rate correspond to an unequal level of marital fertility, or are imputable to the varying degree of precision of birth statistics or, finally, may be imputable to differences in the sex-age-marital status distribution of the population. The data for 1864 show, in fact, a higher proportion of married fertile women in the south than in the north; it is impossible, however, to know whether the same situation prevailed fifty years before. Assuming that the sex-age-marital status distribution of the 1815-1819 population was the same as in 1864, we have computed an index of marital fertility, standardized by age (I_g), for the south and the north, shown below together with the birth rate. If our assumption is correct, regional differences in birth rate are due to differences in the sex-age-marital status composition of the popu-

[11] *Ibid.*, p. 211.

[12] *Ibid.*, p. 206.

Table 2. Population and Births in Six Portuguese Provinces, 1801 and 1815-1819

Provinces	House-holds	Popu-lation	Inhabi-tants per house-hold	Birth rate	Sex ratio at birth	Found-lings per 100 births
		1801, ecclesiastical subdivisions				
Minho	246,329	953,972	3.87	34.2	110.8	-
Tras-os-Montes	20,900	77,676	3.72	29.3	103.1	-
Beira	223,793	881,004	3.94	32.6	104.6	-
Estremadura	149,356	572,403	3.83	32.4	103.5	-
Alentejo	80,932	288,200	3.56	37.9	102.1	-
Algarve	28,214	100,158	3.55	44.2	105.3	-
Portugal	749,524	2,875,413	3.84	33.9	105.7	-
		1801, geographic subdivisions				
Minho	190,544	737,606	3.87	33.0	-	-
Tras-os-Montes	67,881	262,161	3.86	30.8	-	-
Beira	228,048	892,762	3.91	30.3	-	-
Estremadura	164,934	645,519	3.91	32.2	-	-
Alentejo	80,903	298,166	3.69	36.9	-	-
Algarve	26,194	95,079	3.63	43.5	-	-
Portgugal	758,501	2,931,393	3.86	32.5	-	-
		1815-1819, geographic subdivisions				
Minho	79,386	313,923	3.95	34.3	105.2	9.4
Tras-os-Montes	46,769	185,126	3.96	35.6	108.1	11.1
Beira	87,674	339,413	3.87	36.0	106.7	6.6
Estremadura	111,557	494,593	4.43	35.7	106.0	13.4
Alentejo	50,963	183,180	3.59	44.4	104.3	5.7
Algarve	29,023	113,601	3.91	42.2	110.2	3.4
Portugal	405,372	1,629,836	4.02	36.9	106.3	9.6

Notes: The data for 1815-1819 refer to twenty-four of the forty-four *comarcas*, including 53 percent of the total population. The sex ratio for 1815-1819 excludes foundlings.

lation; regional differences in marital fertility are, therefore, small. This result would also suggest that the differences in the birth rates between the two areas are real, and do not derive from an uneven coverage of the statistics.

Area	*Birth rate*	*Marital fertility (I_g)*
North[a]	35.2	.809
South[b]	43.3	.822
Portugal[c]	36.9	.795
South as percent of north	123.0	101.600

[a] Minho, Tras-os-Montes, Beira
[b] Alentejo, Algarve
[c] including Estremadura.

The data reported in Table 2 show also that the sex ratio at birth—at least for the whole country—was normal, around 1.06. Finally, the proportion of foundlings, around 10 percent of the total, is almost equal to the proportion of illegitimate births recorded at the turn of the century. In the city of Lisbon this proportion was well over 25 percent, a pattern that remained almost unchanged until recent times.

2.3. *Further Statistical Evidence for the Nineteenth Century*

We have noted before that the first modern census was taken in 1864, while the modern organization and collection of vital statistics on a continuing basis started over 20 years later in 1886. Before this date the evaluation of vital rates has to be made on the basis of the existing scanty and discontinuous evidence. In Table 3[13] we have reported the birth rates for Portugal from the beginning

[13] The data on births are drawn from the following authors: 1801, Travassos; 1815-19, Balbi-Franzini; 1843 and 1849-51, A. de Oliveira Marreca (*Parecer e memoria sobre un proyecto de estatística*, presented at the Academia Real de Ciências); 1864, 1871-75, G. Pery (adjusted data, *Statistique du Portugal et des colonies*, Lisbon, 1878); 1886-92 and 1900-04, official sources. The birth rates for 1811 and 1878 have been obtained through stable techniques, combining the census age distribution with the intercensal rate of growth (1801-20 and 1864-78). The age distribution for 1811 is reported in Estatística de Portugal, *Censo no 1° de janeiro 1864*, Lisbon, 1868, p. xvi, and is drawn from the *Investigador Portuquez em Inglaterra*, Vol. I, pp. 106, 112. The data derived from the works of Marreca and Pery are reported in Instituto Nacional de Estatística, *Recenseamento da população, 1940*, Vol. XXIV-XXV, p. 20, Table 20.

Table 3. Portuguese Birth rates during the Nineteenth Century

Year	Birth rate	Index numbers Average = 100
1801	33.9	101.7
1811	33.2	99.6
1815-1819	36.5	109.5
1843	31.2	93.6
1849-1851	32.3	96.9
1864	33.6	100.8
1871-1875	32.7	98.1
1878	33.8	101.4
1886-1892	33.9	101.7
1900-1904	32.1	96.3
Average	33.3	100.0

of the nineteenth to the beginning of the twentieth century, gathering together data on population and births derived from different sources. It is almost impossible, with the information at our disposal, to evaluate the reliability of the series reported in Table 3. The precision of our data depends both on the completeness of birth registration (baptisms) and on the completeness of the enumerations of the population. We know that both elements are probably more or less defective, but we do not know to what extent. However, two facts have to be pointed out. The first is that the various approximate figures reveal a constant level of natality, mostly around 33 per thousand[14] during the century; the

[14] A. Almeida Garrett, "Dos problemas a natalidade," *R.C.E.D.*, n. 3, p. 68, reports the birth rate for the city of Porto and for the Porto region for 1785-87 and for 1880-89:

	1785-87	*1880-89*
Porto	38.3	38.3
Porto region	37.3	35.5

The data for 1785-87 are derived from the work of A. Rebelo da Costa,

second is that the correction of the birth rate at the end of the nineteenth century, raises its value by a mere 4 percent (see 3.3.). Moreover, estimates of the birth rate at several dates during the nineteenth century, derived from the application of stable population techniques, give results almost identical to the average for the entire period 1801-1904.

It is safe to draw the following conclusions:

(1) The birth rate seems constant throughout the century, although it is probably underestimated by at least 4 percent.

(2) The average level must be regarded as fairly low for predecline times, and comparable only to the levels prevailing in England and Wales and in the Scandinavian countries before the onset of the secular decline of fertility.

(3) The relatively low level of the birth rate may be explained by the combination of a moderate marital fertility rate with a low propensity to marriage.

Descripção topographica e historica da cidade do Porto, Porto, 1788. Even for the city and for the area of Porto, the data show a remarkable stability of the birth rate from the end of the eighteenth to the end of the nineteenth century.

CHAPTER 3: Population Statistics and Population Growth During the Last Century

3.1. *The Censuses*

The census of 1864 is the first with modern characteristics; the count was nominative, simultaneous, and individually taken. Another census followed in 1878, and subsequently a law was passed in 1887 that required a census to be taken every ten years, beginning in 1890.[1]

In Portugal we encounter the same problems that exist in the censuses of other countries with a low level of social development. The age distribution is strongly affected by misreporting of ages, the distorting influence of which has been very strong until relatively recent times. The distortion is strong enough to influence five-year age groups as well as the distribution by single years; in general, the population enumerated in the groups including ages terminating in zero is significantly enlarged at the expense of those including ages terminating in five. For the fecund age groups encompassing an age terminating in zero (including the groups 20-24 through 50-54), we have computed the average percent overestimate in the census enumerations from 1864 to 1960:[2]

1864	+ 17.1	1920	+ 1.6
1878	+ 15.8	1930	+ .9
1890	+ 4.9	1940	− .8
1900	+ 4.8	1950	− 1.7
1911	+ 4.9	1960	− .8

[1] For a survey of the census characteristics, 1864 to 1960, see J. T. Montalvão Machado, "No centenario do I censo populacional Português," in *R.C.E.D.*, n. 16, 1965.

[2] For each age group (C_{20-24}, C_{30-34} etc.) we have computed the ratios $C_{20-24}/.50(C_{15-19}+C_{25-29}) = k_{20}$; $C_{30-34}/.50(C_{25-29}+C_{35-39}) = k_{30}$ etc. The average of k_{20}, k_{30}, k_{40} and k_{30}, or $\bar{k}$, has been divided by the corresponding average of the four k'—or $\bar{k}'$—obtained from a stable population having the same expectation of life and birth rate of the Portuguese population. The value of $\bar{k}'$, however, is always very close to unity, independent of the various levels of mortality and fertility. The ratio k/k' only exceptionally equals unity, although this value is approached, because of the irregularities in the age composition imputable to fluctuation of vital rates, migration, wars, etc.

The distortion of the first two censuses, of 1864 and 1878, is very strong and probably would affect any computation based on the age distribution. The three censuses at the turn of the century—1890, 1900, and 1911—although revealing conspicuous improvements, still show the existence of errors in the age distribution. From 1920 on, the situation is almost normal.

The age distribution of the infant population is even more gravely defective. The census population in the first year of life is substantially understated and inferior in number to the enumerated population between 1 and 2 years of age. The latter group probably includes many children who should be listed in the first. The same phenomenon happens in the two first five-year age groups (0-4 and 5-9); the first group is underenumerated, and part of its components are "transferred" to the older age group.[3]

The extremely low cultural and educational level of the Portuguese population is probably a primary factor in the poor accuracy of the first census counts. In 1878, approximately 4/5 of the population over 6 years of age could neither read nor write. This proportion decreased very slowly to 2/3 in 1920 and to 1/2 in 1940. Illiteracy, as is well known, tends to reduce the precision of an operation (such as a census) which, although not complex, does require accuracy of response.

3.2. *Vital Statistics*

The collection and publication of vital statistics began only in 1886, although in 1878 a law had created an "optional" civil register.[4] Let us say that the registration of deaths was unreliable, by admission of the official sources, until the beginning of this century. Death statistics were based on burial permissions granted by the civil authorities who frequently failed to compile the statistical forms, and the results are accordingly gravely defective until 1890.[5] The coverage was complete only in the sense that

[3] See Appendix.

[4] Almeida Garrett, "Os problemas da natalidade," in *R.C.E.D.*, n. 2, pp. 33ff.

[5] R. Jorge, *Demographia e hygiene da cidade do Porto*, Porto, 1899, pp. 221-23.

every area of the country compiled the required statistics, the accuracy of which, however, left much to be desired.

For births, the data were generally drawn from parish registers. In 1886, for instance, only the districts of Évora, Portalegre, and Ponta Delgada, and the *concelhos* of Lisbon and Porto had reliable civil registers, while the information for the rest of the country was derived from the books of baptisms.[6] Although all live-born children had to be baptized, there is little doubt that a fraction of the newborn who died in the first hours or in the first days of life were not registered because they had not been baptized. Many were declared as stillbirths, in order to avoid the formalities of burial permission. Since birth statistics, until 1911, were predominately registration of baptisms and not of births, it is certain that registration of births was incomplete.[7] It is difficult, however, to estimate the degree of inaccuracy of registration, but two facts have to be taken into account. The first is that the newborn was, in the opinion of Almeida Garrett, baptized within two weeks in the countryside and in the villages, and within the first month in the large cities.[8] Assuming that all infants were baptized at the average age of ten days, and that those dead before then were all excluded from the count (which is not the case), not more than 4 percent of all births would be excluded from the count (with a level of infant mortality around 250 per thousand).[9] The second element is the estimate, made by Jorge, of the number of infant deaths declared as stillbirths ("false stillbirths") in the city of Porto. During the years 1893-1897, the total number of live births was 26,628, of which 347 were "false stillbirths," or 1.3 percent of the total.[10] It is safe to assume that the proportion of live births not registered because of early death varies between a minimum of 1 and a maximum of 5 percent.

[6] Direcção Geral do Commercio e Industria, *Movimento da População, primeiro anno, 1887*, Lisbon, 1890 (see the Introduction).

[7] Jorge, *op. cit.*, p. 258. Almeida Garrett, *op. cit.*, p. 37.

[8] Almeida Garrett, *op. cit.*, p. 36.

[9] When infant mortality is around 250 per thousand, certainly no more than 15 percent of all deaths under one year take place before the tenth day, or about 4 percent of total deaths.

[10] Jorge, *op. cit.*, p. 260.

In 1911, according to a law passed on February 18, civil registration of births became obligatory beginning April 1. Registration had to occur within one week, a period prolonged to one month in 1912. During that year, and for part of the following, those children born before the law and not registered were entered in the registers; in fact, the statistics show that the number of births registered in 1911 was at least 1/5 higher than the average number for 1908-1910.[11] After 1911, birth statistics attained a good level of accuracy, and the calculation of fertility rates does not require an adjustment.

The completeness of birth registration can be judged by various indices. The sex ratio, only slightly influenced by abortion and stillbirths, tends to be practically constant through time, with little territorial variability, at the average level of 105-106 male births for every hundred female. Every notable variation from this level, when the number of observations is sufficiently large,[12] is suspect, and almost certainly derives from incomplete registration of births of one sex or the other. Usually, female births suffer more than male births from underregistration, as can be seen in frequent instances, in the existence of an abnormally high sex ratio. In the following table, we show the districts where the sex ratio exceeded, in various periods, the limit of 108, a level indicating almost certainly a sizeable underregistration of females:

1888-1892		*1901-1904*		*1909-1913*	
Aveiro	108.2	Bragança	111.2	Ponta Delgada	108.6
Beja	110.6	Guarda	108.6		
Bragança	109.3	Leiria	108.1		
Évora	115.5	Lisbon	112.1		
Guarda	110.4	Viana do Castelo	109.5	*1918-1922*	
Horta	110.3	Horta	112.3	Bragança	108.9

In the two periods preceding 1911, six provinces exceeded the limit of 108, evidently the consequence of an incomplete registration.

[11] The average annual number of births, 1907-10, was 178.4 thousand; the average for 1912-15 was 196.4; the number of registered births in 1911 was 230.0, against an estimated level of 187.4 (or 178.4 + 196.4/2), or 22.3 percent more.

[12] Only the sex ratio of Horta is based on a number of births slightly below 10,000.

3.3. *Controls and Adjustments*

Birth statistics may be compared with the data from census enumerations as a way of detecting underregistration. The procedure is based on the obvious fact that in a closed population, the enumerated population at a certain date and under a certain age—for instance, under 10 years—derives from the births which occurred in the 10 years preceding the census date. With the help of a record of deaths distributed by age or of an estimate of the level of infant mortality, it is very easy to estimate the number of births from census data. The comparison between "estimated" and "registered" births gives the measure of the underregistration of births, at least relative to the enumerated population under 10 years old.

Two conditions are necessary in order to make such a procedure a valid estimate of completeness of registration. First, it is necessary that the census statistics be reasonably accurate both in completeness of coverage of the child population and in precision of age reporting. In the second place, it is necessary to have a reliable evaluation of the level of mortality. Neither of the two conditions is completely realized in Portugal. Census statistics present a strongly biased age distribution, as we have previously pointed out; moreover, there are no reliable evaluations of the level of mortality. Before 1920, deaths were not distributed by age, and the first "official" life table was compiled only in 1940.

Taking this into account, the correction of birth statistics through any "indirect" method becomes quite difficult. At the national level we have attempted an estimate of underregistration through backward projection of the census population under 10 years of age and comparison with the births registered in the 10 years before the census. The coefficients for the backward projection of the census population have been derived from the Princeton model life tables (South).[13] The appropriate life table has been selected by finding the model life table that would yield the rate of natural increase and the death rate of the decade preceding the census.

[13] A. J. Coale and P. Demeny, *Regional Model Life Tables and Stable Populations*, Princeton, 1966.

Births thus estimated are subsequently compared with births effectively registered during the same period. Shown below are the results of the comparison (also see Appendix):

Years	*Estimated births*	*Registered births*	*Percent difference*
1891-1900	1,669,560	1,601,028	−4.1
1902-1911	1,838,039	1,841,950	+0.2
1911-1920	1,789,477	1,904,408	+6.4

The data lend themselves to the following considerations:

(1) Underregistration is evident, although not strong, in the last decade of the nineteenth century. It is almost certain that also in the first decade of this century births were underregistered, although the computation presented above shows a slight excess of registered overestimated births. Underregistration in the decade from 1901 to 1910 is obscured by the inclusion in the statistics of 1911 of about 40,000 births that occurred in the preceding years, but that were registered only after the new law on compulsory registration had been passed in 1911.

(2) In the decade from 1911 to 1920, registered births largely exceeded estimated births, or, in other words, census data seem to be less exact and reliable than registered vital events. It may be, however, that the discrepancy between registered and estimated births is also imputable to the effects of the exceptional mortality due to the epidemic of influenza at the end of the decade—an epidemic not properly estimated as far as its effects on the younger population were concerned (see Appendix).

(3) The underregistration of 4.1 percent at the end of the nineteenth century may be regarded perhaps as too low to be accepted. This may be so, but it is also true that the birth rate estimated through stable techniques—assuming the age distributions of 1890 and 1900 and the rates of increase of 1878-1890 and 1890-1900—yields a birth rate very close to that obtained by correcting registered births for the above mentioned level of underregistration.

(4) The comparison between registered and estimated births tends to ascertain the consistency between the two sets of statistics, but neither of the two terms of the comparison can be considered completely exact and reliable. In the case of Portugal, it appears that accuracy increases more rapidly in birth statistics than in census data (at least in the very young age groups). Besides, it is a common experience for many southern European countries (Italy, Spain, and also France) that vital statistics were more reliable than census enumerations. In these countries it may be dangerous and misleading to attempt to estimate births starting from census statistics.

Taking these points into consideration, we have proceeded to the correction of the birth statistics from 1886 to 1904, assuming for the whole period an underregistration of 4.1 percent. A different correction factor, however, has been estimated for every district, since the proportion of the births omitted from the statistics varied from district to district. The criteria for the calculation of these correction factors are illustrated in the Appendix. The correction factors run from a minimum of 1-2 percent (islands, Castelo Branco, Aveiro, Guarda, Viana do Castelo) to a maximum of 8 percent for Lisbon and some provinces of Tras-os-Montes and Alentejo.

3.4. *Population Settlement, Growth, and Redistribution*

Several factors, such as climate, topography, access to the sea and waterways, land distribution, and political history, have determined the varying pattern of population settlement over the Portuguese territory. Following Ribeiro,[14] four principal types of demographic settlement can be individuated:

(1) Type "Minhoto," of Minho, part of Beira and of Douro littoral, with a rural population evenly spread through land long cultivated for a wide variety of traditional crops; the population density is very high.

[14] Ribeiro, "Portugal," *op. cit.*, pp. 194-97.

(2) Type "Transmontano," of Tras-os-Montes and Beira Transmontana, with a general pattern of concentration of the population in rural villages and centers, and with a low density.

(3) Type "Alentejano," of Alentejo, southern Ribatejo and part of Beira Baixa; the population is agglomerated in large rural villages, separated one from another by large, almost deserted areas. This type of settlement is associated with a pattern of extensive cultivation of cereals and with the prevalence of latifundia. Density is very low.

(4) Type "Estremeño," of Estremadura, part of Beira and Ribatejo, and Algarve. There is tendency toward demographic concentration in some urban areas, combined with a remarkable dispersion of the population throughout the territory. Population density is high.

The various types of settlement correspond also to substantial differences in regional demographic dynamics. The Minhoto and Transmontano type of settlement is associated with a traditional propensity to emigrate, induced in the first case by the excessive density and fragmentation of land and, in the second, by the unfavorable living conditions of the Transmontanos. The type Estremeño is characterized by rapid urbanization (associated with internal immigration) and population growth.

In Table 4, data are given on the development of the resident population in the various districts from the first official census in 1864 to 1960. In this and in the following tables we have reported the districts in geographical order, working from east to west and from north to south. In fact, we have followed historical precedent indicating development from the interior toward the coast in a direction from the northcentral area toward the south, and we have adopted that orientation in ordering the territorial districts of the country. Subsequently, we shall see also how certain demographic phenomena are in close relationship with this northeast-southwest orientation.

Analysis of Table 4 reveals, first of all, how the demographic

Table 4. Population of the Districts, 1864-1960

(000 of inhabitants)

Districts	1864	1878	1890	1900	1911	1920	1930	1940	1950	1960
1. Bragança	161	172	180	185	192	170	187	214	228	233
2. Vila Real	218	232	239	241	246	235	256	291	319	325
3. Viana do Castelo	204	212	214	219	232	230	233	261	279	278
4. Braga	317	328	340	358	383	378	414	488	546	597
5. Porto	420	468	549	599	681	707	806	941	1,054	1,193
6. Guarda	215	233	252	265	274	259	260	296	308	283
7. Viseu	366	389	399	410	422	411	442	469	495	482
8. Aveiro	252	270	292	306	340	347	392	433	483	525
9. Castelo Branco	160	177	206	217	244	242	262	305	325	317
10. Coimbra	282	308	328	339	368	360	377	416	439	434
11. Leiria	177	197	220	242	270	283	310	358	396	405
12. Santarém	202	227	255	283	322	335	378	426	460	462
13. Lisbon	349	415	498	566	682	743	903	1,055	1,222	1,383
14. Portalegre	98	106	115	126	144	151	165	189	200	188
15. Évora	102	114	122	129	150	156	179	210	222	219
16. Setúbal	92	102	115	134	166	186	233	270	326	377
17. Beja	135	149	159	165	195	203	243	278	291	277
18. Faro	177	204	230	257	276	271	296	320	328	315
19. Angra	74	72	72	73	70	67	71	78	86	96
20. Horta	65	64	59	55	50	46	49	53	55	49
21. Ponta Delgada	111	128	125	129	123	118	135	156	177	182
22. Funchal	110	132	134	150	170	180	212	249	270	269
Portugal	4,287	4,669	5,103	5,447	5,999	6,080	6,802	7,755	8,510	8,889

development of the various districts—on the continent and in the islands—has been differentiated during the last century. The population has quadrupled in the districts of Lisbon and Setúbal, has diminished in that of Horta, and has increased by only 1/3 in Viana do Castelo, Guarda, and Viseu. As a rule, the population has increased very rapidly in the five districts along the coast from Porto to Lisbon (Porto, Aveiro, Coimbra, Leiria, and Lisbon). The increment has been slightly more than the national norm in the districts south of the Tagus and much less in the other districts, namely those to the interior, north of the Tagus. The differential demographic increase of these areas can be seen concisely in the following table:

Areas	*Population* 1864	*Population* 1960	*Percent of distribution* 1864	*Percent of distribution* 1960	*Percent of change* 1960/1864
Coast from Porto to Lisbon	1,480	3,940	37.7	47.5	+166
Other districts north of the Tagus	1,843	2,977	46.9	35.9	+ 62
Districts south of the Tagus	604	1,377	15.4	16.6	+128
Continent	3,927	8,294	100.0	100.0	+111

It is worth noting that the rapid expansion of the coastal area is in part due to the pull of the urban center of Lisbon and in part also to a favorable evolution of the birth and death rates. The rather slow growth of the other provinces of the north is, in contrast, the consequence of a permanent migratory deficit which has been compensated for only partially by the high birth rate. This is the area that more than any other has contributed to the demographic growth of Brazil and to the emigration to other European countries in recent decades. Finally, in the districts south of the Tagus, emigration has always been negligible (with the exception of some areas of the Algarve), and the moderate growth has been the result of an especially marked drop of the natural increase of the population. The average emigration rates for the 1900-1960 period are reported in Table 5, and reveal the impressive regional differentials in the propensity to emigrate: the maximum level on

Table 5. Average Emigration Rates[a] by District, 1900-1960

Bragança	8.4	Santarém	.9
Vila Real	6.8	Lisbon	.7
Viana do Castelo	4.2	Portalegre	.3
Braga	3.9	Évora	.1
Porto	3.7	Setúbal	.1
Guarda	7.0	Beja	.3
Viseu	7.5	Faro	2.0
Aveiro	7.3	Angra	8.6
Castelo Branco	1.0	Horta	7.4
Coimbra	5.3	Ponta Delgada	10.3
Leiria	3.5	Funchal	9.5
	Portugal	4.7	

[a] Annual number of emigrants per 1,000 population at mid-period.

the continent is attained by the Transmontanos districts, Aveiro and Coimbra; the minimum can be found in Alentejo.[15] The emigration rates are also very high in the islands.

The demographic densities of the various areas present considerable contrasts (see Table 6). All the districts that border on the sea to the north of the Tagus have a high density, with a minimum, in 1960, of 110 inhabitants per km.^{2} in Coimbra. All districts of the "interior," north of the Tagus, have rather low population densities ranging between 36 in Bragança and 77 in Vila Real.

15 For an appraisal of regional emigration, see J. de Souza Bettencourt, "El fenomeno de la emigración Portuguesa," in *Revista internacional de sociologia*, 1959-60, n. 68, n. 69.

Table 6. Population Density of the Districts, 1864-1960

(Inhabitants per km.^{2})

Districts	1864	1878	1890	1900	1911	1920	1930	1940	1950	1960
1. Bragança	25	26	28	28	29	26	29	33	35	36
2. Vila Real	52	55	56	57	58	55	60	69	75	77
3. Viana do Castelo	97	100	101	104	110	109	110	124	133	132
4. Braga	116	120	125	131	140	139	152	179	200	219
5. Porto	184	205	241	262	298	310	353	412	462	523
6. Guarda	39	42	46	48	50	47	47	54	56	51
7. Viseu	73	78	80	82	84	82	88	94	99	96
8. Aveiro	93	100	108	113	126	128	145	160	179	194
9. Castelo Branco	24	27	31	32	36	36	39	45	48	47
10. Coimbra	71	78	83	86	93	91	95	105	111	110
11. Leiria	52	57	64	71	79	83	90	104	115	118
12. Santarém	30	34	38	42	48	50	57	64	69	69
13. Lisbon	126	150	180	205	247	269	327	382	443	501
14. Portalegre	17	18	20	22	24	26	28	32	34	32
15. Évora	14	15	17	17	20	21	24	28	30	30
16. Setúbal	18	20	22	26	32	36	45	52	63	73
17. Beja	13	15	16	16	19	20	24	27	28	27
18. Faro	35	40	45	50	54	53	58	63	65	62
19. Angra	103	102	102	104	99	95	101	111	123	137
20. Horta	86	83	76	72	65	60	65	69	72	65
21. Ponta Delgada	132	151	148	152	146	140	160	185	210	216
22. Funchal	139	166	168	189	213	226	267	313	339	337
Portugal	67	51	56	60	66	66	74	85	93	97

This is clearly related to the unfavorable morphological characteristics for settlement in a great part of the area. To the south of the Tagus, population density is still lower, even though the level nature of the terrain would be considered suitable for settlement. The lowest population density can be found in Beja (27) and the highest, in Setúbal (73).

Summing up, the regional demographic growth of Portugal fits in well with the general tendencies of the Iberian peninsula since the eighteenth century; these are tendencies of a centrifugal nature, which increase the weight of the peripheral areas with respect to the central ones, and Portugal is no exception to this general rule.[16]

3.5. *The Balance of Births and Deaths*

Before getting into a detailed analysis of nuptiality and fertility, it is important, in our opinion, to take a look at the general tendencies of the vital rates during the 80-year period from 1886 to 1965. The balance of births, deaths, and migration is reported in Table 7; the various computations are based exclusively on unadjusted official data, and are therefore affected by the not negligible distortion and incompleteness of official enumerations, especially in the first two or three decades. Since deaths, more than births, are the subject of incomplete registration, it is possible that net migration is overestimated in the first decades.

The data of Table 7 call for a few comments. In the first place, let us note the varying impact of net migration, always negative over the 80 years considered here: the net loss through emigration is high and increasing until the period 1912-1920; it is reduced to almost nothing in the 30-year period between 1921 and 1950; and it attains its highest levels in the last fifteen years. It is important to note that, if we exclude the anomalous case of Ireland, Portugal is the country with the highest rate of net emigration in western Europe, with a net loss approaching, in the last 80 years, 2 million people.

[16] M. Livi Bacci, "Fertility and Nuptiality Changes in Spain from the Late 18th to the Early 20th Century," Part 2, in *Population Studies*, Vol. XXIII, 2, 1967, p. 213.

Table 7. The Balance of Births, Deaths, Migration, 1886-1960

Period	Live births	Deaths	Natural increase	Census population beginning of the period	Estimated population end of the period	Census population end of the period	Net migration	Population at mid period	Birth rates	Death rates	Migration rates	Rates of increase: Natural	Rates of increase: Actual
	(1)	(2)	(1)−(2) =(3)	(4)	(4)+(3) =(5)	(6)	(6)−(5) =(7)	½(4+6) =(8)	(1):(8). 1000=(9)	(2):(9). 1000=(10)	(7):(8). 1000=(11)	(9)−(10) =(12)	(12)−(11) =(13)
1886-90	818.6	554.8	263.8	4,841.6	5,105.4	5,049.7	− 55.7	4,945.7	33.10	22.44	−2.25	10.66	8.41
1891-00	1,601.0	1,112.9	488.1	5,049.7	5,537.8	5,423.1	−114.7	5,236.4	30.57	21.25	−2.19	9.32	7.13
1901-11	2,012.8	1,263.4	749.4	5,423.1	6,172.5	5,960.1	−212.4	5,691.6	32.15	20.18	−3.39	11.97	8.58
1912-20	1,714.4	1,288.8	425.6	5,960.1	6,385.7	6,033.0	−352.7	5,996.5	31.77	23.88	−6.53	7.89	1.36
1921-30	2,058.3	1,247.9	810.4	6,033.0	6,843.4	6,825.9	− 17.5	6,429.4	32.01	19.41	−0.27	12.60	12.33
1931-40	2,013.6	1,184.9	828.7	6,825.9	7,654.6	7,722.2	− 67.6	7,274.0	27.68	16.29	−0.93	11.39	10.46
1941-50	2,025.2	1,237.4	787.8	7,722.2	8,510.0	8,441.3	− 68.7	8,081.7	25.06	15.31	−0.85	9.75	8.90
1951-60	2,092.1	991.3	1,100.8	8,510.0[a]	9,610.8	8,889.4[a]	−721.4	8,699.7	24.05	11.51	−8.29	12.54	4.25
1961-65	1,077.3	486.5	590.8	8,889.4[a]	9,480.2	9,171.3[b]	−308.9	9,030.3	23.85	10.77	−6.84	13.08	6.24

[a] Resident population; for other dates, present population

[b] Estimated resident population

As for mortality, the slowly declining trend puts Portugal far behind other countries; the death rate of almost 20 per thousand in 1921-1930 was attained, on the average, nearly 30 years before by the western European countries, according to the computations of Sundbärg. The expectation at birth of a life span of 66 years, in 1960, indicated the worst health conditions in all Europe, with the possible exception of Albania.

Finally, the birth rate remained almost unchanged between 1886-1890 and 1921-1930, around 31-33 per thousand; it declined in the following two decades but attained a new plateau, around 24-25 per thousand in the last 25 years. Here, again, Portugal was far behind the western European countries, whose birth rates had fallen, in the great majority of cases, below 24 per thousand before or immediately after the First World War. Even the Italian birth rate had fallen below 24 per thousand in the early 1930s, while Spain has consistently remained below this level since the end of the civil war.[17]

[17] In Spain, however, the birth rate has remained almost unchanged since 1940, although remaining below the Portuguese levels. The Spanish birth rate was, in 1941-43, 20.8 per thousand; in 1948-53, 20.9 per thousand, and in 1958-63, 21.3 per thousand.

CHAPTER 4: Trends and Differentials in Portuguese Nuptiality

4.1. *Nuptiality in Portugal as a Whole*

The analysis of nuptiality and of its changes through time is a necessary preliminary to the study of fertility. In western Europe in the nineteenth century the age at which marriage occurred and the proportion of persons remaining single at the end of their fecund life influenced fertility at least as much as differences in the rate at which married women bore children.

As a first step, it is important to have an exact quantitative knowledge of the terms of the problem. To give an example, in 1878 the proportion of women of childbearing age who were currently married was, in the district of Faro, over 75 percent higher than that reported in the district of Horta. Ignoring illegitimacy and differences in age composition, and assuming an equal marital fertility in the two populations, the birth rate of the first should also exceed the birth rate of the second by 75 percent.

The censuses after 1864 show the population distribution according to age, sex, and marital status; measures of the propensity toward marriage can, therefore, readily be derived from the census data, enabling us to follow the trends in nuptiality during the last century.

Three different indices of nuptiality have been computed:

(1) The weighted proportion married in the female population of childbearing age (15 to 49 years). This measure, symbolized by I_m, is designed to describe nuptiality in terms of its potential effect on fertility.[1] It depends on the average age at marriage, on the proportion of women who never get married, and on the frequency of widowhood and remarriage.

(2) The proportion married among women 20-24 years of age. This measure is closely correlated with the average age at

[1] See note 1, Chapter 5.

marriage, and is a good index of the tendency to get married early or late.

(3) The proportion of single women between 50 and 54 years of age, which can be regarded as an index of definitive nubility. This is an index of the proportion of women who do not marry before the end of the childbearing age and who, therefore, do not contribute to the marital fertility of the population.

It is obvious that these indices are contaminated by the misreporting of ages pointed out in 3.1., particularly when misreporting affects in a different way the married and the unmarried population. Besides the measures derived from census data, current statistics of marriages are another source for the study of nuptiality which may usefully supplement the indices presented above.

In Table 8, we have reported several measures of nuptiality, 1864 to 1960, for the whole Portuguese population. The first consideration is that many of the indicators point towards a substantial stability of nuptiality until 1940, followed by a sudden increase in the last two decades. The marriage rate, mostly between 6.5 and 7 per thousand until 1930, rapidly increases, reaching 8.3 in 1958-1962; the proportion married, I_m, oscillating between .45 and .48 from 1878 to 1940, suddenly climbs to .51 in 1950 and to .56 in 1960. It is important to point out that the proportion married is, until 1940, substantially lower than in the Mediterranean countries (Italy, Spain, Greece).[2] The increase in the propensity toward marriage goes along with a growing proportion of married females in the 20-24 age group (around 30 percent at the end of the nineteenth century; 41 percent in 1960), indicating a falling age at marriage (around 24 years in the last decades).

Perhaps even more interesting considerations can be derived from the statistical series of the proportion of single females, 50 to 54 years of age. The proportion of females who never marry at

[2] Here are the values of I_m for Italy, Spain, and Greece. Italy, 1901 = .549, 1931 = .512; Spain, 1900 = .559, 1930 = .564; Greece, 1900 = .632, 1928 = .566.

Table 8. Portuguese Nuptiality, 1864-1960

Years	Marriage rate[a]	Index of the proportion married I_m	Percent unmarried 50-54		Percent married 20-24	
			M	F	M	F
1864	--	.424	14.7[b]	21.7[b]	12.8[c]	26.1[c]
1878	7.00	.452	13.0[b]	20.2[b]	16.0[c]	31.4[c]
1890	6.91	.456	14.3	22.2	14.3	29.6
1900	6.83	.460	13.0	21.4	15.2	30.4
1911	6.59	.471	11.5	18.9	16.5	30.9
1920	7.63	.455	11.4	18.2	15.9	29.1
1930	6.70	.474	--	16.8	16.4	30.8
1940	6.71	.476	--	16.8	18.6	33.5
1950	7.84	.513	10.4	16.7	16.0	34.3
1960	8.29	.556	--	16.0	19.0	41.0
		Index numbers, 1864 = 100[d]				
1864	--	100.0	100.0	100.0	100.0	100.0
1878	101.3	106.6	88.4	93.1	125.0	120.3
1890	100.0	107.5	97.3	102.3	111.7	113.4
1900	98.8	108.5	88.4	98.6	118.7	116.5
1911	95.4	111.1	78.2	87.1	128.9	118.4
1920	110.4	107.3	77.6	83.9	124.2	111.5
1930	97.0	111.8	--	77.4	128.1	118.0
1940	97.1	112.3	--	77.4	145.3	128.4
1950	113.5	121.0	70.7	77.0	125.0	131.4
1960	120.0	131.1	--	73.7	148.4	157.1

a Notes refer to the following years: 1875 (Pery's data), 1888-1892, 1898-1902, 1909-1913, 1918-1922, 1928-1932, 1938-1942, 1948-1952 and 1958-1962.

b 51-55 age group.

c 21-25 age group.

d For marriage rates, 1888-1892 = 100.

all is very high, even in comparison with other European countries, reaching a level of over 22 percent in the latter part of the nineteenth century, and slowly decreasing to 16 percent in 1960. This would indicate that at the end of the last century between 1/4 and 1/5 of the female population was excluded from the process of legitimate reproduction; a higher proportion could be found at the turn of the century only in Ireland, generally considered an anomalous case-limit within the western European pattern of nuptiality.[8] Portuguese society had apparently put in action rather efficient checks of a Malthusian type that severely limited the number of births. These restrictions have been slightly eased only in the last decades; they clearly explain the reasons for the relatively low level of the birth rate during the predecline period.

4.2. *Aspects of Regional Nuptiality*

The behavior of the Portuguese population is far from being homogeneous as far as marriage habits are concerned. Deep economic and social contrasts differentiate regional societies also as far as the marriage patterns are concerned. We will devote this section to the statistical analysis of regional nuptiality and will attempt an interpretation in the following one.

Tables 9 and 10 contain the values of the index of the proportion married (I_m) by districts, 1864 to 1960, and the corresponding index numbers (1890 = 100). Geographical variations in the value of I_m for 1864 and 1960 and in the change in value over this period are presented in Figures 2 and 3. The tendency to a substantial increase of I_m, more rapid in recent times, is common to all districts north of the Tagus, but cannot be found in the south. This differential trend, however, seems to be related to the uneven levels of I_m prevailing at the end of the last century. In 1864, 1878, and 1890, the lowest values of I_m could be found in the north—Viana do Castelo, Vila Real, Viseu, Braga, Aveiro—and in the

[8] In 1900, the highest proportions of single women aged 45 to 49 in Western Europe could be found in Ireland (29 percent), Portugal (20 percent), and Sweden (19 percent). See J. Hajnal, "European Marriage Patterns in Perspective," in *Population in History*, edited by D. V. Glass and D. E. C. Eversley, London, 1965, p. 102, Table 2.

Table 9. Weighted Index of the Proportion of Married Females

15-49 Years, I_m, 1864-1960

Districts	1864	1878	1890	1900	1911	1920	1930	1940	1950	1960
1. Bragança	.440	.448	.438	.438	.468	.432	.448	.494	.518	.562
2. Vila Real	.388	.407	.389	.405	.427	.408	.445	.471	.503	.540
3. Viana do Castelo	.345	.358	.354	.357	.361	.347	.374	.388	.431	.469
4. Braga	.372	.387	.403	.418	.428	.396	.429	.463	.470	.511
5. Porto	.386	.447	.461	.453	.457	.430	.460	.475	.508	.557
6. Guarda	.459	.486	.489	.483	.509	.487	.511	.533	.553	.562
7. Viseu	.383	.412	.401	.400	.430	.416	.457	.482	.519	.544
8. Aveiro	.381	.421	.418	.428	.447	.423	.455	.494	.543	.594
9. Castelo Branco	.492	.518	.525	.518	.524	.491	.516	.551	.574	.575
10. Coimbra	.406	.426	.429	.436	.463	.444	.477	.497	.524	.572
11. Leiria	.474	.441	.474	.514	.484	.484	.519	.515	.545	.586
12. Santarém	.506	.470	.501	.518	.499	.524	.561	.551	.574	.615
13. Lisbon	.510	.460	.471	.468	.441	.445	.432	.422	.476	.552
14. Portalegre	.556	.550	.563	.552	.570	.539	.551	.561	.570	.606
15. Évora	.496	.510	.498	.497	.534	.497	.509	.467	.497	.536
16. Setúbal	-	-	-	-	-	-	.489	.448	.515	.382
17. Beja	.534	.582	.566	.538	.571	.538	.484	.449	.447	.466
18. Faro	.541	.601	.565	.560	.566	.549	.537	.525	.576	.566
19. Angra	.337	.376	.418	.461	.510	.490	.506	.527	.593	.649
20. Horta	.353	.341	.379	.391	.473	.452	.478	.530	.573	.622
21. Ponta Delgada	.477	.481	.474	.417	.565	.568	.556	.535	.550	.601
22. Funchal	.448	.514	.485	.504	.523	.475	.487	.503	.467	.486
Portugal	.424	.452	.456	.460	.471	.455	.474	.476	.513	.556

Table 10. Index Numbers of I_m, 1864-1960
(1890=100)

Districts	1864	1878	1890	1900	1911	1920	1930	1940	1950	1960
1. Bragança	100.5	102.3	100	100.0	106.9	98.6	102.3	112.8	118.3	128.3
2. Vila Real	99.7	104.6	100	104.1	109.8	104.9	114.4	121.1	129.3	138.8
3. Viano do Castelo	97.5	101.0	100	100.9	102.0	98.0	105.7	109.6	121.8	132.5
4. Braga	92.3	96.0	100	103.7	106.2	98.3	106.5	114.9	116.6	112.7
5. Porto	83.7	97.0	100	98.3	99.1	93.2	99.8	103.0	110.2	120.8
6. Guarda	93.9	99.4	100	98.8	104.1	99.6	104.5	109.0	113.1	114.9
7. Viseu	95.5	102.7	100	99.8	107.2	103.7	114.0	120.2	129.4	135.7
8. Aveiro	91.1	100.7	100	102.4	106.9	101.2	108.9	118.2	129.9	142.1
9. Castelo Branco	93.7	98.7	100	98.7	99.8	93.5	98.3	105.0	109.3	109.5
10. Coimbra	94.6	99.3	100	101.6	107.9	103.5	111.2	115.9	122.1	133.3
11. Leiria	100.0	93.0	100	108.4	102.1	102.1	109.5	108.6	115.0	123.6
12. Santarém	101.0	93.8	100	103.4	99.6	104.6	112.0	110.0	114.6	122.8
13. Lisbon	108.3	97.7	100	99.4	93.6	94.4	91.7	89.6	101.1	117.4
14. Portalegre	98.8	97.7	100	98.0	101.2	95.7	97.9	99.6	101.2	107.6
15. Évora	99.6	102.4	100	99.8	107.2	99.8	102.2	93.8	99.8	107.6
16. Setúbal	-	-	100	-	-	-	-	-	-	-
17. Beja	94.3	102.8	100	95.1	100.9	95.1	85.5	79.3	79.0	82.3
18. Faro	95.8	106.4	100	99.1	100.2	97.2	95.0	97.9	107.9	100.2
19. Angra	80.6	90.0	100	110.3	122.0	117.2	121.1	126.1	141.9	155.3
20. Horta	93.1	90.0	100	103.2	124.8	119.3	126.1	139.8	151.2	164.1
21. Ponta Delgada	100.6	101.5	100	88.0	119.2	119.8	117.3	112.9	116.0	126.8
22. Funchal	92.4	106.0	100	103.9	107.8	97.9	100.4	103.7	96.5	100.2
Portugal	93.0	99.1	100	100.9	103.3	99.8	104.0	104.4	112.5	121.9

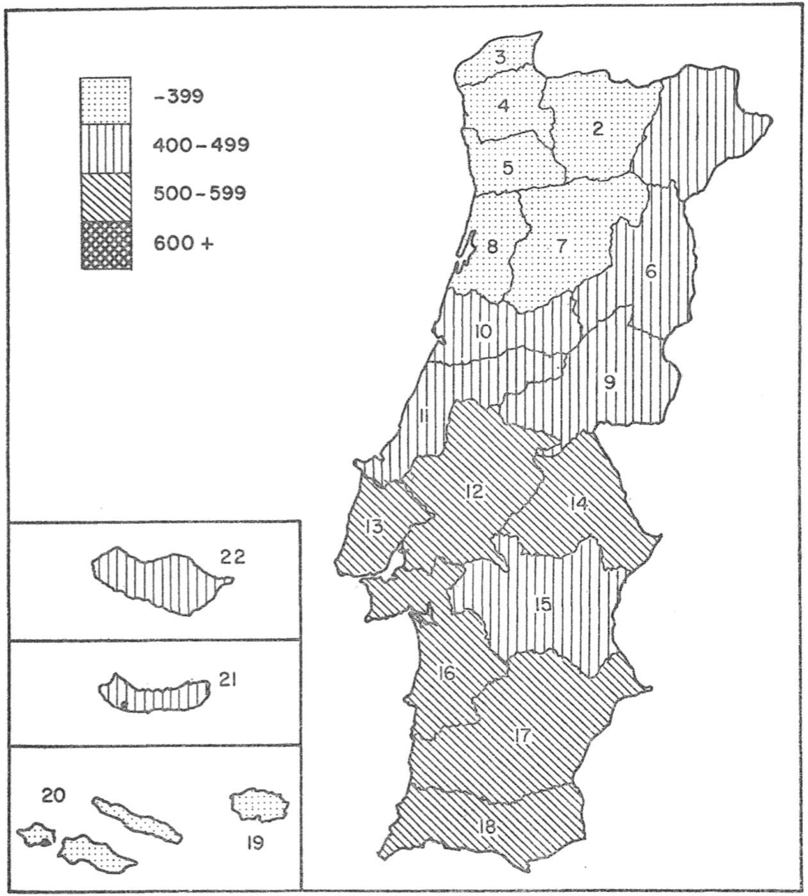

Figure 2a. Weighted index of proportion married, I_m, 1864

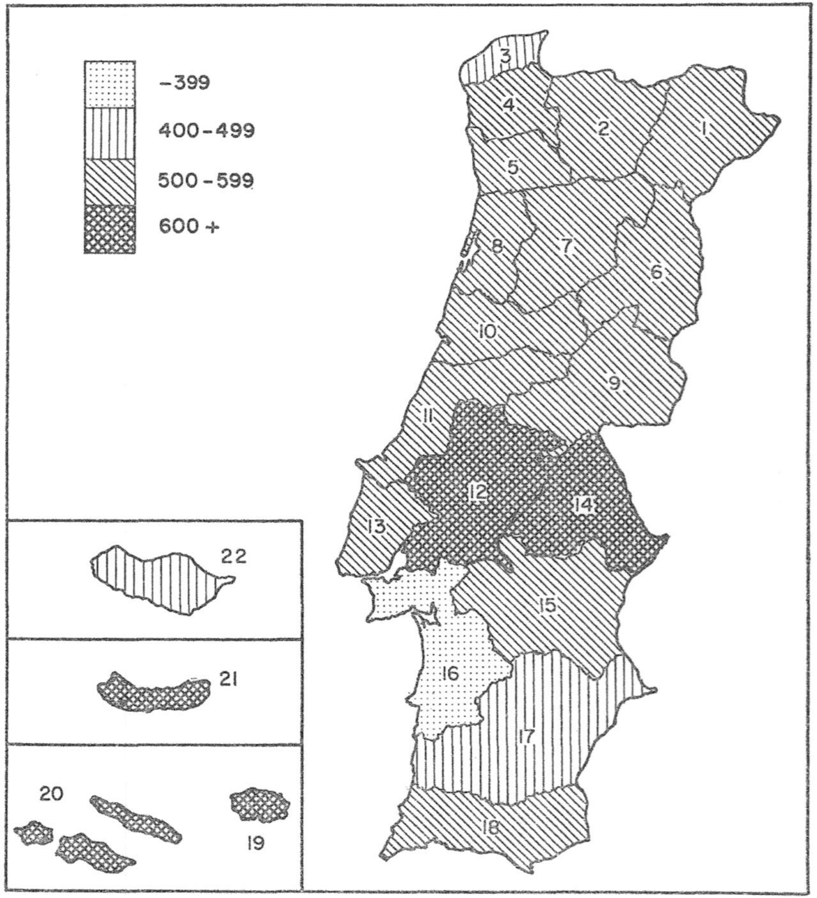

Figure 2b. Weighted index of proportion married, I_m, 1960

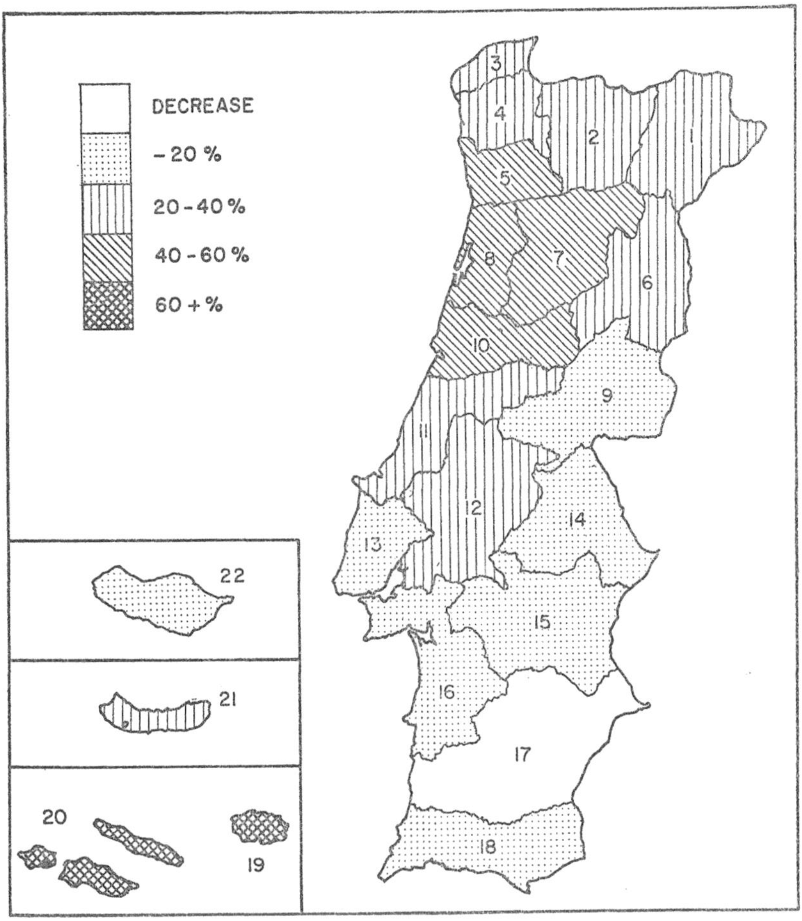

Figure 3. Percentage increase in the weighted index of proportion married, I_m, 1864-1960

Azores, with levels below or around .400. The highest levels could be found in the districts of Alentejo and Algarve, and also in Santarém and Castelo Branco; in many of these districts I_m has remained, over the last century, almost constant (Faro, Portalegre, Évora), or has substantially decreased (Beja). In 1960, the highest nuptiality could be observed in Santarém, Portalegre, and in the Azores (over .600) and the lowest in Beja and Viana do Castelo (.47).

It is interesting to note that the sharp increase in the propensity toward marriage has changed the geography of nuptiality. The correlation coefficient between the values of I_m in 1890 and 1960 is nearly 0 (+.001), indicating no relation whatsoever between the situations of 1890 and of 1960. This finding is in sharp contrast with the experience of Spain and Italy, where the territorial differentials in nuptiality have remained almost unaltered through time.

The second indicator of nuptiality, the proportion married at 20-24 years of age, is shown in Table 11; it is, as we have said, a good substitute for the mean, modal, or median age at marriage. The proportion of married women in this age group increases for the whole country from 26 to 41 percent over the last century, indicating a substantial decrease of the age at marriage. Turning the attention to the districts, it can be observed, as expected, that the highest incidence of young married women occurred, in the nineteenth century, south of the Tagus; the lowest to the north (Viana do Castelo, Braga, and Coimbra). In 1960, these territorial differentials had been totally cancelled and partially inverted; the correlation coefficient between 1864 and 1960 is —.226.

Table 12, presenting the median age at first marriage of males and females in 1950, supplements the data of Table 11.[4] As expected, the districts with lower age at marriage are also those with the higher proportion married at age 20-24.

The third indicator of nuptiality, perhaps the most interesting one from a sociological point of view, is the proportion remaining single at age 50-54 (Table 13). We have already commented upon the national data, and will not repeat ourselves; as usual, however, the national average obscures the diversity of the territorial situations which vary a great deal. The proportion of single women at age 50-54 never falls below 10 percent, but in a number of districts it often exceeds 30 percent. The highest levels can be found in the Minho and, in general, in the districts north of the Mondego river, with the exception of Guarda. In this area, the

[4] The mean age at marriage has remained almost constant during the last two decades, between 24-25 years for females and 26-27 for males. On nuptiality, see J. J. Paes Moraes, "Tábuas de extinção de solteiros para 1940 e 1950," in *R.C.E.D.*, n. 9. *Idem.* "Alguns aspectos demograficos da população Portuguesa," in *Estudos of the Instituto Nacional de Estatística*, n. 18, Lisbon, 1960.

Table 11. Proportion Married, Female Population 20-24 Years, 1864-1960

Districts	1864	1878	1890	1900	1911	1920	1930	1940	1950	1960
1. Bragança	30.5	31.7	26.8	28.3	30.2	28.5	30.9	33.4	34.9	39.4
2. Vila Real	23.4	28.5	24.7	25.9	27.6	26.9	30.1	32.0	34.7	37.3
3. Viano do Castelo	15.5	19.0	16.9	18.9	19.2	17.0	22.0	21.2	24.3	36.7
4. Braga	19.1	24.8	23.6	27.5	26.1	22.7	24.8	-	30.0	34.4
5. Porto	22.9	34.2	34.1	31.8	31.7	27.5	31.2	31.2	35.9	43.6
6. Guarda	28.2	34.3	29.6	31.0	32.6	30.0	32.1	34.6	36.2	39.0
7. Viseu	20.8	26.7	22.7	23.2	26.0	26.0	29.6	32.3	34.9	39.4
8. Aveiro	20.6	26.9	27.0	25.8	28.2	26.0	30.1	34.0	39.6	49.9
9. Castelo Branco	32.6	38.2	34.0	32.2	33.6	29.3	31.7	35.1	37.6	39.6
10. Coimbra	19.6	23.5	23.1	23.0	26.6	25.4	28.5	29.9	33.5	42.2
11. Leiria	22.2	22.7	24.4	36.6	26.0	27.4	30.4	31.0	34.9	38.7
12. Santarém	29.9	28.9	28.3	30.3	30.4	32.6	36.7	37.0	38.4	44.8
13. Lisbon	30.5	33.3	33.2	32.5	29.8	30.8	27.8	25.7	31.1	40.9
14. Portalegre	44.2	43.9	41.2	39.1	41.0	35.5	35.8	38.4	38.1	42.6
15. Évora	34.9	39.2	34.7	35.9	38.8	30.5	34.5	28.5	31.0	34.4
16. Setúbal	-	-	-	-	-	-	35.8	31.1	39.1	45.0
17. Beja	40.1	48.5	40.4	39.2	42.6	36.3	27.2	21.3	22.8	25.0
18. Faro	42.7	49.1	43.6	39.4	41.1	39.2	36.1	35.2	42.2	45.1
19. Angra	17.1	27.0	28.7	35.1	38.0	35.7	38.0	37.2	44.7	53.7
20. Horta	16.3	22.3	26.4	25.5	35.9	33.5	38.0	37.5	44.4	48.3
21. Ponta Delgada	30.9	37.8	33.3	33.7	45.8	45.7	43.3	33.5	34.8	46.1
22. Funchal	33.7	41.2	35.4	35.5	40.0	33.4	37.5	34.3	30.2	43.7
Portugal	26.1	31.4	29.6	[30.4]	30.9	29.1	30.8	33.5	34.3	41.0

Table 12. Median Age at First Marriage, by District, 1950

	F	*M*		*F*	*M*
Bragança	23.1	26.2	Santarém	23.0	25.2
Vila Real	23.1	25.6	Lisbon	24.0	26.8
Viana do Castelo	24.3	26.2	Portalegre	22.9	25.6
Braga	23.4	24.9	Évora	23.6	27.1
Porto	23.0	24.8	Setúbal	22.6	25.9
Guarda	23.0	25.1	Beja	24.6	27.7
Viseu	23.1	25.2	Faro	22.4	25.7
Aveiro	22.4	24.3	Angra	22.8	26.7
Castelo Branco	22.9	24.8	Horta	22.5	26.5
Coimbra	23.2	25.1	Ponta Delgada	23.2	26.5
Leiria	23.4	25.1	Funchal	22.8	25.5
			Portugal	23.2	25.6

proportion of women remaining single is almost always above 20 percent until 1911-1920. South of the Tagus river and in Santarém and Castelo Branco, the proportion of unmarried women is substantially lower, between 10 and 15 percent.

Long-term changes in the proportion remaining single follow a pattern geographically differentiated. In the provinces of the north the proportion remaining single tends to decrease slightly, while in the south there is an increase; by 1960 the gap between the two areas has narrowed. Lisbon, geographically to the south, shows a high proportion remaining single (around 20 percent); but here the consequences of the selective immigration of females are at work, creating a situation of unbalance in the sex structure common to many urban agglomerates.

On the whole, the deep contrasts separating the north from the south tend to cancel off as time goes by; the factors underlying the different behavior of these areas cannot be easily identified; nevertheless we will devote the next section to the effort of advancing some tentative interpretations.

4.3. *Some Factors of Nuptiality Differentials*

The interpretation of the deep regional differentials in nuptiality is certainly very complex, since there are many factors likely

Table 13. Proportion Single, Females 50-54 Years

1864 - 1960

Districts	1864	1878	1890	1900	1911	1920	1930	1940	1950	1960
1. Bragança	21.3	18.1	20.7	-	18.6	19.9	18.5	17.0	14.0	13.0
2. Vila Real	25.2	24.3	27.8	-	25.2	25.3	22.4	21.0	17.7	15.4
3. Viana do Castelo	27.8	27.7	31.5	-	30.6	29.7	29.2	28.9	28.2	25.2
4. Braga	26.9	27.2	31.4	-	26.3	24.7	22.0	23.5	20.6	17.9
5. Porto	24.0	23.2	26.1	-	21.1	19.7	18.9	19.9	19.4	17.2
6. Guarda	-	15.2	16.8	-	14.0	12.8	11.8	13.0	11.6	11.5
7. Viseu	24.9	22.7	26.3	-	24.1	24.3	21.0	21.9	18.7	16.5
8. Aveiro	23.4	22.8	24.9	-	21.8	19.9	20.8	20.2	19.0	17.0
9. Castelo Branco	15.7	14.1	13.8	-	11.2	12.1	9.2	9.7	10.0	9.0
10. Coimbra	20.2	19.2	21.1	-	19.2	19.2	16.7	17.7	15.9	15.1
11. Leiria	26.5	11.6	12.8	-	10.1	10.4	9.6	11.3	10.4	10.0
12. Santarém	13.7	12.3	13.2	-	9.6	9.8	8.8	10.0	9.5	9.5
13. Lisbon	22.2	20.9	20.2	-	18.1	18.1	20.2	21.6	20.3	19.8
14. Portalegre	13.1	13.3	14.3	-	10.4	9.6	9.5	9.6	9.1	10.6
15. Évora	12.3	16.3	16.2	-	15.7	16.2	13.5	12.9	13.4	15.4
16. Setúbal	-	-	-	-	-	-	12.3	17.2	18.0	19.2
17. Beja	11.3	11.5	13.1	-	11.5	10.4	9.7	11.6	13.5	18.2
18. Faro	11.0	9.0	10.4	-	9.8	8.8	8.0	9.2	10.8	12.8
19. Angra	20.2	26.4	32.7	-	25.1	22.6	17.6	18.6	14.8	12.5
20. Horta	23.7	32.1	35.9	-	33.2	26.5	21.7	24.4	19.6	17.4
21. Ponta Delgada	14.8	16.8	18.3	-	18.3	17.4	12.9	10.6	9.1	10.1
22. Funchal	16.0	21.5	19.5	-	15.7	14.4	13.3	17.9	16.7	15.3
Portugal	21.7	20.2	22.2	(21.4)	18.9	18.2	16.8	18.1	16.7	16.0

to influence the marriage habits of the population. But even after a superficial appraisal of the characteristics of the regional societies, two aspects can be easily singled out as having a deep influence on nuptiality. The first important one is the heavy emigration from almost all districts of the north; it is, as we have previously pointed out, an emigration of males which has deeply altered the sex structure of the population and, therefore, affected the opportunities for marriage of the female population. The second, maybe even more important, factor of nuptiality differentials consists of the varying forms of ownership and distribution of land, and of the transmission of property from one generation to the following.

It is important to bear in mind, before proceeding any further in our analysis, that the two factors outlined above are mutually related, since emigration is itself a consequence of the régime of land property and distribution; if we treat the two aspects separately, it is only for the sake of presenting our arguments more clearly.

The first step is to explain the reasons for the deep nuptiality differentials—between north and south—existing in the nineteenth century and maintained, even if in an attenuated form, until the end of the First World War. Emigration, mainly overseas, has always been very strong from the north of the country—in all districts north of the Tagus, as a matter of fact, with the exception of Lisbon, Santarém, and Castelo Branco. In the latter districts and in the south, emigration has always been rare—with the exception of Faro—because of the low density and of the need of manpower in the large estates of Alentejo and also because of the pull of the urban agglomerate of Lisbon—all factors that have, on the other hand, caused emigration from other areas of the country. Emigration has deeply altered the sex structure of the population; females exceeded males in all censuses until 1930 by 9 to 11 percent, this disproportion being imputable almost exclusively to the areas of emigration and to the young age groups. It is obvious that the permanent emigration of many young men has lessened the opportunities for women to marry, and made female celibacy a common phenomenon.

Emigration cannot be the sole explanation for the very low nuptiality of the north, and this for several reasons. The first is that nuptiality has increased in the last 20 years or so in spite of the tremendous wave of emigration that started—after a long period of stagnation—in the late forties, revealing clearly that factors other than migration are at work in determining nuptiality trends. The second is that the proportion of males remaining single—although never attaining the levels reached by the female population—was fairly high in the nineteenth century, reaching 15 percent in the 50-54 age group. There is no doubt that for the young males remaining in the country there were plenty of marriage opportunities, given the very favorable (to them) sex structure; as a consequence, the high incidence of celibacy cannot be explained by emigration only.

The other explanation of nuptiality differentials can be found in the régime of land property and distribution. In the north where the average size of properties was very small the land was increasingly fragmented in every generation.[5] The land of the smallest owners would be equally subdivided between the heirs in ridiculously small shares. But the fragmentation of the farms of larger size often had to be avoided in order to preserve the economical size of the farm unit; then the older son would inherit the land, and the cadets either would be given an equal value in money or kind,[6] if the family were rich, or would be left with their hands empty, ready for emigration or for the cloister, and very often destined to remain unmarried. Until the nineteenth century, the institution of the *Morgado*, the practice of entailing land to the older son, provided a legal support for the preservation of the unity of properties. In the words of Villier, "in spite of the abolition of the Morgado . . . the use of entailing the family property to the elder son still survives. The others piously bow and leave, searching elsewhere their fortune."[7] The same situation could be

[5] Ribeiro, "Portugal," *op. cit.*, pp. 172ff.

[6] Dias, *op. cit.*, pp. 118-120.

[7] Villier, "Portogallo," *op. cit.*, p. 131.

found in the eighteenth and nineteenth centuries in northern Spain, and particularly in Galicia and Asturias.[8]

In the often cited study of Descamps, the opinion of Andrade Borges, who has studied the Barroso area (Tras-os-Montes), is reported: "It is only when a family owns enough land to be self-sufficient, that the property, instead of being subdivided (among the heirs) is left unshared, at the price of the celibacy of many. This requires a strong education based on the father's authority, and developing the attachment to traditions, the love for labour and for the family, sobriety and religiosity."[9] Emigration opens a chance for men, and Descamps observed of Tras-os-Montes that "now the majority of young men who cannot get married in their country, choose to leave. It is not so for girls, who often vow themselves to remain unmarried under the spell of certain religious mysticism."[10] The interrelations between marriage habits, land ownership, and inheritance are shown by Descamps for the whole north of Portugal, in the Barroso as in Ponte do Lima, in Braga as in Maia.[11]

The very high number of vocations in the Minho, already pointed out by Balbi in the early nineteenth century,[12] certainly has roots in the deep religiosity of the people, but can also be related to the opportunities that the Church offered young men and women left without subsistence and excluded from marriage. Customs restrictive of marriage have survived until relatively recent times in Tras-os-Montes, such as the prohibition for the girls of the Serra de Gerce to marry persons coming from other villages.[13]

All these impediments and restrictions to marriage do not exist in the south. In Alentejo, where large estates prevail, emigration is unknown and by far the largest share of the rural population is formed by farm laborers; they certainly do not have problems of

[8] M. Livi Bacci, "Fertility and Nuptiality Changes in Spain," *op. cit.*, pp. 221-22.

[9] Descamps, *op. cit.*, p. 4.

[10] *Ibid.*, p. 53.

[11] *Ibid.*, pp. 4, 70, 80, 96.

[12] Balbi, "Essai statistique," *op. cit.*, Vol. II, p. 10.

[13] Descamps, *op. cit.*, p. 17. Villier, *op. cit.*, pp. 137ff.

inheritance to solve.[14] Women very rarely are economically active, while in the north, either because of the high incidence of nubility, because of emigration of males, and because of the prevalent type of varied cultivations, they are frequently employed in the fields (but also in industry, textiles, for instance). In 1900, if we rely on census statistics—and we have no valid reasons to suspect their reliability in this respect—seven women for every ten men were economically active in the districts of the Minho, against a proportion of two to ten for those of Alentejo.

During this century we have seen an increase of nuptiality in the north and its stagnation in the south; the deep contrasts existing in the nineteenth century have been partially cancelled. The reasons for the increase of nuptiality in the north are not clear, but they are probably related to the abolition of the Morgado with the civil code of 1867; to the fading of certain customary restrictions pointed out earlier; to increasing mobility; to a substantial, even if slow, industrialization which has freed part of the rural population from ancient patterns of behavior. The stagnation of nuptiality in the south can be ascribed not only to its relatively high starting levels, but also to the diffusion of a certain reluctance to get married. Montalvão Machado observes how the young people resort less and less to marriage, particularly in certain areas of western Alentejo (Alcacér do Sal, Grandola, S. Tiago do Cacem, Odemira) where illegitimate births often exceed the legitimate.[15] Descamps, again, reports that in Alentejo, "after the Republic, religious practices have been abandoned in many villages, particularly in the south and in the west. People do not get married in the Church; often they do not even perform the civil marriage, because it costs 180 escudos."[16] Further on he says that in the *concelho* of Grandola "marriage is rare; two young people start living together,

[14] The predominance of wage workers in the south goes back to remote times; see Silbert, "Le Portugal" *op. cit.*, p. 822, who gives several examples for the eighteenth century. In Serpa, in 1793, over 1,233 persons engaged in agriculture while 938 were wage earners.

[15] J. T. Montalvão Machado, "Alguns aspectos da natalidade," in *R.C.E.D.* no. 10, p. 134ff.

[16] Descamps, *op. cit.*, p. 193.

sometimes they part, sometimes they spend together all life. When they have two or three children they perform the civil marriage."[17]

People of Algarve and Alentejo, it is well known, are not very religious; in Setúbal or Évora only 40 to 50 percent of the marriages were performed with, or followed by, a religious rite (1950). A large fraction of the population declared itself atheist in various censuses. Family ties, not enforced by a deep attachment to religion, are less strong than in the north; divorce exists, but it is expensive and many people believe that it is more practical to live together without marriage and part freely when the time comes.

Given this particular mentality, and given the increasing frequency of irregular "menages," it is not surprising that nuptiality has remained constant, or has even dramatically declined, as in Beja. It is possible also that the changes in the marriage legislation after the Concordat have diverted more people from getting indissolubly married.

[17] *Ibid.*, p. 123.

CHAPTER 5: A Descriptive Outline of Regional Fertility

5.1. *A Century of Portuguese Fertility*

Official statistics of vital events make it possible to follow the fertility of the Portuguese districts from 1890 to 1960. As we have said previously, the data until the beginning of this century have been adjusted in an effort to eliminate underregistration of births.

The measures of fertility adopted in this chapter are exclusively period measures derived from the combination of vital and census statistics. The information on fertility that can be derived from the 1940, 1950, and 1960 census surveys will be examined at length in the following chapter.

For the descriptive analysis of regional fertility, we have computed a series of standardized indices, where the standard fertility schedule is derived from the age-specific fertility rates of the Hutterites' marriages of 1921-1930.[1] We have computed an index of general fertility (I_f), an index of legitimate fertility (I_g), and an index of illegitimate fertility (I_h) such that

$$I_f = I_g \cdot I_m + I_h \cdot (1 - I_m).$$

The F_i values of the standard fertility schedule employed for the computation of the various indices of fertility are derived from the experience of the Hutterites' marriages, 1921-1930, and assume for the different age groups the following values: 15-19=.300; 20-

[1] The indices of fertility and nuptiality, standardized by age, adopted in our study, can be defined as follows: Let us designate by the symbols f_i, g_i, and h_i respectively the total, legitimate, and illegitimate births per woman in the ith age interval; by w_i, m_i, and u_i respectively the number of total, married, and unmarried women in the ith age interval, and by F_i the births per woman in the ith age interval in the standard population (married Hutterites, 1921-30). We obtain the following expressions:

$$I_f = \frac{\Sigma f_i w_i}{\Sigma F_i w_i} \quad (1); \qquad I_g = \frac{\Sigma g_i m_i}{\Sigma F_i m_i} \quad (2); \qquad I_h = \frac{\Sigma h_i u_i}{\Sigma F_i u_i} \quad (3); \qquad I_m = \frac{\Sigma F_i m_i}{\Sigma F_i w_i} \quad (4)$$

where the numerators of (1), (2), and (3) are respectively the actual number of total legitimate and illegitimate live births. The standard schedule is reported in Table 14. See A. J. Coale, "Factors Associated with the Development of Low Fertility, An Historic Summary," *World Population Conference 1965*, Vol. II, p. 205.

24=.550; 25-28=.502; 30-34=.667; 35-39=.406; 40-44=.222; 45-49=.061. To the above mentioned indices of fertility we have added a corrected index of marital fertility (I_g'), designed to eliminate the effects of the unbalance in the sex-structure of the married population induced by migration.

Before undertaking the territorial analysis of fertility trends, it seems worthwhile to outline the trend of fertility for the whole country, from 1864 to 1960 (Table 14). The values for 1864 are

Table 14. Fertility Measure of the Portuguese Population 1864 - 1960

Year	Index of the proportion married (I_m)	Birth rate per thousand	Index of general fertility (I_f)	Index of marital fertility (I_g)	Index of marital fertility corrected (I_g')	Index of illegitimate fertility (I_h)
1864	.424	33.6	.329	.682	.684	(.079)
1878	.452	33.8	.341	.664	.672	(.079)
1890	.457	33.9	.358	.689	.709	.079
1900	.460	32.1	.353	.681	.700	.073
1910	.471	33.5	.344	.636	.674	.083
1920	.455	31.3	.318	.609	.642	.075
1930	.474	30.2	.304	.544	.542	.088
1940	.481	25.0	.257	.453	.463	.076
1950	.513	25.2	.255	.440	.459	.059
1960	.556	24.3	.255	.414	.435	.057
			Index numbers, 1864 = 100			
1864	100.0	100.0	100.0	100.0	100.0	100.0
1878	106.6	100.6	103.6	97.4	98.2	100.0
1890	107.8	100.9	108.8	101.0	103.7	100.0
1900	108.5	95.5	107.3	99.9	102.3	92.4
1911	111.1	99.7	104.6	93.3	98.5	105.1
1920	107.3	93.2	96.7	89.3	93.9	94.9
1930	111.8	89.9	92.4	79.8	79.2	111.4
1940	113.4	74.4	78.1	66.4	68.4	96.2
1950	121.0	75.0	77.5	64.5	67.1	74.7
1960	131.1	72.3	77.5	60.7	63.6	72.2

based on Pery's data for births, while the estimate of the fertility measures for 1878 has utilized the well-known stable techniques of analysis, assuming the Portuguese population "closed" and with approximately constant levels of fertility and mortality.[2] The assumption that the Portuguese population was stable is probably sound for the second half of the nineteenth century; the long-term fertility decline starts after 1910 and, as far as mortality is concerned, we may assume that its change was gradual and slight at that time, as it was in Spain and in Italy. Moreover, although Portugal is a country of ancient emigration, it is only toward the end of the nineteenth century that emigration assumes the characteristics of a mass movement. The fertility indices for the other dates are based on the average number of births registered in the five-year period centered around the census dates.[3]

[2] See note 13, Chapter 2.

[3] The fertility rates reported in Tables 14, 15, 16, 17, and 22, have been obtained as follows: For 1864, the various indices are based on the number of births in 1861, reported in the 1864 census volume, *op. cit.*, p. xvi. The census volume reports the figure of 137,954 births, which, adjusted to 1864, assuming an annual rate of increase of .52 percent (rate of growth of the total population, 1841-64), gives an estimate of 140,161 births for that year. Assuming the same level of illegitimacy as that of 1888-92 (12 percent), the estimated number of legitimate births is 123,341. The estimate of the birth rate for 1878 has been made by employing stable techniques of analysis, combining the census-cumulated age distribution (up to the ages of 15, 25, 35, 45, 55, and 65 years) for males and females separately, with the 1864-78 rate of increase (.61 for males and .63 for females), and taking the median of the six estimates of the birth rate for each sex (32.6 for females and 35.0 for males). The estimated birth rate (33.8 per thousand) has been multiplied by the census population, obtaining the total number of births, from which the number of legitimate births has been obtained.

From 1890, fertility indices are based on registered births, corrected at the beginning as indicated in the Appendix. The exact date of the census enumerations and the years for which the births have been considered are reported below:

Census Date	*Births*
December, 1890	1888-92
December, 1900	1901-04
December, 1911	1909-13
December, 1920	1918-22
December, 1930	1928-32
December, 1940	1938-42
December, 1950	1948-52
December, 1960	1958-62

From 1897 to 1906 the annual publication of demographic data was discontinued. Retrospective data, by district, were published for 1901 and the following years in

The data reported in Table 14 speak for themselves, and it will not take a long time to comment on them. We will try, in the following pages, to outline the principal implications of the data presented in the table; and we will not repeat many of the observations concerning the fertility trends of the whole population when we later examine territorial trends and differentials.

It is interesting to note, in the first place, that the relatively low pattern of nuptiality prevailing at the end of the nineteenth century resulted in a relatively low level of the birth rate and of general fertility. The birth rate of eastern Europe exceeded nearly everywhere the 40 per thousand level; in the Mediterranean countries the birth rate was well above 35 per thousand (36-37 per thousand in Spain and in Italy). The birth rate of Portugal was around 32-33 per thousand, which was as low as or lower than the levels prevailing in England or in the Scandinavian countries before the onset of the secular decline, and which did not resemble the levels prevailing in eastern, central, or southern Europe. The same holds true for general fertility. The decline of both general fertility and the birth rate occurred slowly and was nearly imperceptible until 1930. At this date the two measures had lost only 8-10 percent of the 1864 levels. The largest decline occurred between 1930 and 1940; after 1940 and until 1960 both the birth rate and the general fertility remained nearly constant, at levels which can be regarded as rather high, if compared with the European average. A birth rate of approximately 25 per thousand, such as the Portuguese had in the years around 1960, coupled with a general mortality rate of 10 per thousand, corresponds to a rate of natural increase of 15 per thousand—an increase which in the Mediterranean populations tends to contribute to the typical con-

---

Arquivos do Instituto Central de Higiene, "Tabelas do movimento fisiologico da população de Portugal," Lisbon, 1916. For 1909-12, only the data on total live births were tabulated; legitimate births for 1909-13 have been estimated, applying to the total births of the period the proportion (for each district) of legitimate over total births of 1913. Also for 1928 the number of legitimate births is unknown; the ratio of legitimate to total births, computed for 1929-32, has been extended accordingly to the entire period.

ditions of economic underdevelopment (high emigration, excessive labor force, unemployment, underemployment).

The development of legitimate fertility, as expressed by I_g, follows a rather different course. In the first 40 years of the period taken into consideration—namely until the beginning of this century—marital fertility remained constant, around .68–.69. From the beginning of the century until 1920 there is a slight decrease of I_g, followed by a continuous decline until nowadays. On the whole, the index of marital fertility has decreased over a hundred years by approximately 40 percent, with 3/4 of the decrease concentrated after 1920. If we compare the trend of fertility of Portugal with other European countries, it may be pointed out that marital fertility in the second part of the nineteenth century was relatively low, sharing the situation prevailing in the Mediterranean countries before the onset of the decline, even though I_g was at levels slightly higher than in Spain or in Italy. The situation has been reversed in recent years; in 1960 Portugal had one of the highest rates of marital fertility in Europe, exceeded only by Albania, Ireland, and Yugoslavia, and superior to Holland.[4]

The corrected index of marital fertility, I_g', closely follows the course of I_g, although the decline appears to be weaker and seems to start later in time.

The determination of the period in which an irreversible decline of fertility had started offers an interesting basis for comparing fertility trends in different countries. Several methods could be followed in an attempt to individuate this period. We have used two different criteria: With the first one, we assume that an irreversible process of fertility decline has started once fertility has declined 10 percent below the initial "plateau"; with the second, we select the period in which the index of marital fertility declines below .600. When marital fertility falls below this level, it is almost certain that the population has adopted efficient methods for the control of births, methods which are usually destined for further

[4] M. Livi Bacci, "Sur les régions de l'Europe où la fécondité demeure élevée," *European Population Conference*, Strasbourg, 1966, Vol. I, CDE(66)C6.

diffusion within the population. It is between 1911 and 1920 that I_g falls 10 percent below the 1864 level, while the same decrease is accomplished by I_g' between 1920 and 1930. Both I_g and I_g' fall below the .600 mark between 1920 and 1930.

There is no doubt that Portuguese fertility started its irreversible decline after the end of the First World War, a few decades later than the declines began in Italy and in Spain.

Finally, it has to be noted that the rate of illegitimate fertility is very high, and remains relatively stable until 1940, showing a slight decline thereafter. Comparable levels of illegitimacy can be found only in the countries of central and northern Europe, such as Austria, Eastern Germany, and Sweden, in contrast to the very low illegitimacy prevailing in Spain and Italy.[5]

In the interpretation of fertility trends, we have to bear in mind that illegitimacy has non-negligible weight in the general level of fertility (I_f), a weight varying, for Portugal, between 10 and 13 percent [$I_h \cdot (1-I_m)/I_f$].

5.2. *The Fertility of the Districts*

Table 15 shows the index of general fertility (I_f), by district, from 1890 to 1960. A deeper analysis of territorial trends and differentials will be undertaken in the study of legitimate fertility; therefore, in an effort to avoid repetition, we will limit ourselves to noting the strong contrast existing between the districts of the north—the districts north of the river Mondego numbered 1 to 8 in the tables—and the populations of the valley of the Tagus and of the south (districts south of the Tagus river, numbered 14 to 18 in the tables). In the north of the country, general fertility shows only a slight decrease from the end of the nineteenth century to 1960, a decrease never exceeding 20 percent and, in many instances,

[5] In 1960, the highest proportions of illegitimate births could be found in the following countries: Austria, 13.0 percent; Eastern Germany, 11.4 percent; Sweden, 11.3 percent; Iceland, 25.3 percent; Portugal, 10.0 percent. For Italy, Spain, and Greece the same proportions, in 1960, were respectively of 2.4, 2.3, and 1.2 percent. See United Nations, *Demographic Yearbook 1965*, N.Y., 1966, Table 20, p. 526.

not exceeding 10 percent (Vila Real, Aveiro, Viana do Castelo, Braga: in this last district, I_f shows a substantial increase).

The districts of the Tagus valley (Lisbon, Santarém) and south of the river, all experience a large decrease of the index of general fertility, which falls from 45 to 60 percent below the 1890 levels.

The behavior of the islands is similar to that of the north. In the Azores, for instance, I_f remains at the 1890 levels in two out of three districts. In Tables 16 and 17 we have reported the values of I_g by district and the correspondent index numbers (1890 = 100). The standardized index of marital fertility is the more adequate measure to reveal the start and diffusion of the process of birth control. The consideration and the conclusions that will be drawn on the basis of these tables will be integrated with, and partially modified by, the results of the computations of the corrected index of marital fertility, presented in Table 18.

We shall attempt to summarize below the most important features of the historical series presented in Tables 15-18.

(1) In the districts north of the river Douro (Bragança, Vila Real, Viana do Castelo and Braga) and in the Beira "ultramontana" (Guarda, Viseu), we may note a sharp decrease of marital fertility around 1900 and 1911, followed by a recovery during the successive decades. Such a decrease has to be imputed—at least to a certain extent—to the effects of the particularly heavy emigration at that time. The incessant outflow of migrants, deeply affecting and unbalancing the demographic structure of the population, certainly exerted a depressive influence on marital fertility. The fact that fertility recovered, attaining after 1911 the levels of the end of the nineteenth century, is a clear indication that the decline was not due to voluntary factors. It is not without interest to note that the fertility of the population of southern Italy underwent the same fluctuations between the end of the nineteenth century and the 1920s.[6]

(2) All the districts north of the river Mondego (districts num-

[6] M. Livi Bacci, "Il declino della fecondita della popolazione Italiana nell'ultimo secolo," *Statistica*, Vol. xxv, 3, 1965.

Table 15. Index of General Fertility (I_f) by District, 1890-1960

Districts	1890 (1888-92)	1900 (1901-04)	1911 (1909-13)	1920 (1918-22)	1930 (1928-32)	1940 (1938-42)	1950 (1948-52)	1960 (1958-62)
1. Bragança	.407	.369	.371	.401	.393	.351	.319	.329
2. Vila Real	.358	.345	.334	.354	.409	.328	.346	.352
3. Viana do Castelo	.282	.258	.276	.278	.294	.250	.280	.264
4. Braga	.339	.316	.308	.316	.348	.330	.376	.381
5. Porto	.358	.372	.343	.297	.309	.268	.302	.314
6. Guarda	.407	.398	.390	.373	.336	.318	.299	.265
7. Viseu	.361	.352	.320	.336	.325	.307	.313	.298
8. Aveiro	.337	.356	.333	.313	.310	.284	.297	.307
9. Castelo Branco	.406	.413	.390	.359	.332	.293	.261	.224
10. Coimbra	.316	.282	.281	.271	.251	.220	.219	.218
11. Leiria	.371	.365	.344	.326	.324	.282	.260	.240
12. Santafem	.371	.368	.328	.319	.303	.239	.206	.205
13. Lisbon	.322	.339	.331	.263	.213	.150	.149	.178
14. Portalegre	.338	.392	.388	.355	.315	.247	.203	.189
15. Évora	.347	.395	.385	.352	.320	.252	.207	.175
16. Setúbal	-	-	-	-	.330	.245	.195	.165
17. Beja	.399	.402	.405	.369	.314	.253	.231	.203
18. Faro	.428	.401	.390	.338	.270	.220	.203	.172
19. Angra	.331	.356	.372	.335	.295	.259	.294	.336
20. Horta	.274	.304	.322	.280	.257	.235	.231	.226
21. Ponta Delgada	.388	.360	.431	.423	.351	.306	.324	.388
22. Funchal	.409	.462	.417	.353	.373	.332	.300	.323
Portugal	.358	.353	.344	.318	.304	.257	.255	.255

Table 16. Index of Marital Fertility (I_g) by District, 1890-1960

Districts	1890 (1888-92)	1900 (1901-04)	1911 (1909-13)	1920 (1918-22)	1930 (1928-32)	1940 (1938-42)	1950 (1948-52)	1960 (1958-62)
1. Bragança	.738	.686	.663	.780	.749	.601	.572	.499
2. Vila Real	.714	.686	.646	.708	.758	.567	.598	.590
3. Viana do Castelo	.704	.615	.655	.685	.671	.553	.583	.523
4. Braga	.749	.675	.647	.714	.730	.652	.741	.714
5. Porto	.647	.713	.639	.593	.569	.484	.533	.524
6. Guarda	.760	.770	.721	.725	.622	.568	.522	.460
7. Viseu	.744	.705	.636	.699	.618	.552	.551	.514
8. Aveira	.724	.742	.676	.665	.612	.520	.510	.491
9. Castelo Branco	.735	.766	.719	.702	.619	.512	.441	.378
10. Coimbra	.670	.598	.555	.561	.484	.406	.391	.360
11. Leiria	.738	.669	.658	.618	.439	.478	.429	.376
12. Santarém	.691	.669	.605	.567	.491	.384	.344	.302
13. Lisbon	.552	.559	.540	.427	.332	.230	.236	.260
14. Portalegre	.650	.658	.634	.608	.520	.381	.314	.274
15. Évora	.610	.691	.622	.596	.500	.385	.316	.254
16. Setúbal	-	-	-	-	.445	.314	.246	.197
17. Beja	.639	.672	.640	.602	.542	.429	.375	.300
18. Faro	.702	.654	.617	.544	.419	.317	.284	.250
19. Angra	.711	.725	.713	.659	.563	.472	.480	.503
20. Horta	.650	.726	.651	.593	.507	.415	.383	.405
21. Ponta Delgada	.794	.853	.753	.739	.621	.562	.580	.639
22. Funchal	.800	.786	.784	.729	.757	.643	.623	.649
Portugal	.689	.681	.636	.609	.544	.453	.440	.414

Table 17. Index Numbers of (I_g), 1890 = 100

Districts	1890	1900	1911	1920	1930	1940	1950	1960
1. Bragança	100	93.0	89.8	105.7	101.5	81.4	77.5	67.6
2. Vila Real	100	96.1	90.5	99.2	106.2	79.4	83.8	82.6
3. Viana do Castelo	100	87.4	93.0	97.3	95.3	78.6	82.8	74.3
4. Braga	100	90.1	86.4	95.3	97.5	87.0	98.9	95.3
5. Porto	100	105.8	94.8	88.0	84.4	71.8	79.1	77.7
6. Guarda	100	101.3	94.9	95.4	81.8	74.7	68.7	60.5
7. Viseu	100	94.8	85.5	94.0	83.1	74.2	74.1	69.1
8. Aveiro	100	102.5	93.4	91.9	84.5	71.8	70.4	67.8
9. Castelo Branco	100	104.2	97.8	95.5	84.2	69.7	60.0	51.4
10. Coimbra	100	89.3	82.8	83.7	72.2	60.6	58.4	53.7
11. Leiria	100	90.7	89.2	83.7	59.5	64.8	58.1	50.9
12. Santarém	100	96.8	87.6	82.1	71.1	55.6	49.8	43.7
13. Lisbon	100	101.3	97.8	77.4	60.1	41.7	42.8	47.1
14. Portalegre	100	101.2	97.5	93.5	80.0	58.6	48.3	42.2
15. Évora	100	113.3	102.0	97.7	82.0	63.1	51.8	41.6
16. Setúbal	-	-	-	-	-	-	-	-
17. Beja	100	105.2	100.2	94.2	84.8	67.1	58.7	46.9
18. Faro	100	93.2	87.9	77.5	59.7	45.2	40.5	35.6
19. Angra	100	102.0	100.3	92.7	79.2	66.4	67.5	70.7
20. Horta	100	111.7	100.2	91.2	78.0	63.8	58.9	62.3
21. Ponta Delgada	100	107.4	94.8	93.1	78.2	70.8	73.0	80.5
22. Funchal	100	98.3	98.0	91.1	94.6	80.4	77.9	81.1
Portugal	100	98.8	92.3	88.4	79.0	65.7	63.9	60.1

Table 18. Married Females per 100 Married Males

(De facto population)

Districts	1864	1878	1890	1900	1911	1920	1930	1940	1950	1960[a]
1. Bragança	97.6	98.2	99.1	101.0	103.5	104.6	99.0	100.2	101.9	101.6
2. Vila Real	98.5	99.3	101.2	100.8	107.6	105.9	103.1	102.6	101.9	102.9
3. Viana do Castelo	98.8	105.8	109.7	108.2	112.1	113.5	114.3	113.0	111.1	114.2
4. Braga	102.6	102.9	103.4	103.8	106.3	109.1	104.0	103.8	104.5	106.0
5. Porto	103.3	104.0	103.4	103.7	107.9	106.4	105.0	103.7	104.2	103.7
6. Guarda	100.2	100.2	101.8	103.4	109.0	103.7	111.1	104.7	104.6	104.3
7. Viseu	100.7	103.3	105.2	106.7	114.1	113.3	110.7	109.3	106.7	106.3
8. Aveiro	105.9	108.2	109.4	109.1	114.2	112.9	112.8	107.2	108.3	106.9
9. Castelo Branco	100.1	99.2	97.5	100.6	101.4	103.1	101.5	99.0	101.0	101.5
10. Coimbra	102.3	104.5	106.4	109.8	114.9	111.8	109.7	107.4	107.1	105.2
11. Leiria	101.4	103.0	102.5	103.8	108.1	105.6	104.8	103.8	104.3	102.7
12. Santarém	100.0	99.7	98.5	101.5	99.8	102.3	100.1	101.7	102.5	112.1
13. Lisbon	92.6	93.6	93.3	95.0	94.5	97.2	95.5	96.0	98.8	100.5
14. Portalegre	96.4	98.8	102.5	100.6	101.2	102.2	93.7	99.6	100.7	100.0
15. Évora	99.2	99.2	99.4	98.2	100.5	101.2	100.1	98.9	101.2	99.5
16. Setúbal	-	-	-	-	-	-	95.0	95.9	99.2	100.6
17. Beja	98.5	99.0	97.4	99.2	98.7	100.7	97.4	97.5	99.9	99.4
18. Faro	103.5	101.8	99.2	100.6	104.7	103.6	107.0	102.3	103.7	103.3
19. Angra	102.8	102.1	103.1	101.5	104.6	102.3	100.9	98.9	101.6	101.8
20. Horta	105.5	105.5	106.2	102.9	105.1	103.2	95.7	99.4	102.4	104.5
21. Ponta Delgada	102.5	101.7	102.5	102.1	105.4	103.3	104.3	101.5	102.5	105.9
22. Funchal	100.2	99.8	102.0	100.6	103.5	104.5	102.4	105.7	114.1	113.1
Portugal	150.3	101.2	101.5	102.5	105.3	105.2	103.3	103.3	106.4	103.5

[a] De jure population.

bered from 1 to 8 in the tables) experienced a rather light fertility decline; in 1960 the index of marital fertility was still close to .500 (over .700 in the district of Braga) and the average decline from the 1890 levels was around 25 percent. A similar situation can be found in the islands—Azores and Madeira—where the overall decline has been rather modest.

(3) In the districts of the valley of the Tagus, and south of this river (districts 12-18), on the other hand, fertility declined earlier and more rapidly than in the north, falling to levels between .200 and .300. It is worth pointing out that the fertility of the south of Portugal had attained in the 1950s levels which are among the lowest on record, as low, for example, as in central and northwestern Italy in the years of lowest fertility after 1950. The overall decline in these districts is between 50 and 65 percent.

(4) The districts of Castelo Branco, Coimbra, and Leiria represent, in a certain sense, the transition between the prolific north and the neomalthusian south.[7] In these districts, however, fertility declines rapidly after 1920, reaching levels, in 1960, between .36 and .38.

Summing up, the data indicate a vivid contrast between the north and the south. The decline of fertility seems to follow the geographic order which we have given to the districts, from east to west and from north to south. In Table 16, there is a close inverse relationship between the level of legitimate fertility and the rank of the districts. Whether this is a mere coincidence or the effect of systematic regional influences will be discussed further on.

5.3. *The Impact of Migration*

Table 18 contains the values of the ratio between the total number of married women (F_c) and married men (M_c) in the various

[7] The districts of the center do not have a particular social or economic unity, but they represent, for many aspects, areas where the transition from the north to the south takes place. Latifundia are, for instance, common in the districts of Castelo Branco and Santarém (moreover, about ½ of these districts lie south of the Tagus); fragmented properties are frequent in Coimbra and Leiria.

districts 1864 to 1960. This ratio should be around 100 (F_c/M_c .100) in the absence of abnormal factors causing the separation of couples. When, as happens in many districts of Portugal, an intense emigration—primarily of males—takes place, this ratio tends to increase to well over 100. This means that a certain proportion of married females (approximately equal to 100 F_c/M_c-100) is not subjected to the risk of conceiving a legitimate child. These women should be eliminated, therefore, from the computation of the fertility rates, and this can be done by multiplying the ratio of married females to married males by the legitimate fertility rate

$$I_g' = I_g \,.\, (F_c/M_c)$$

on the assumption that the ratio F_c/M_c, computed on the total married population, does not vary from age to age. This assumption, as the reader can clearly see, is not exact because the sex-unbalance caused by emigration usually affects the young more than the old age groups and, therefore, the more fecund rather than the less fecund women. Thus, the correction factor F_c/M_c is an underestimate.[8]

We have reported in Table 18 the values of the ratio F_c/M_c . 100, which reveals the profound effects of emigration on the sex-structure of the population, particularly in the districts of the north. In Tables 19 and 20 and in Figures 4 and 5, the effects of emigration on fertility are partially corrected by computation of I_g' (and corresponding index numbers); the depression of I_g in 1900 and 1911 is, at least partially, eliminated.

Even so, the general picture of the territorial development of legitimate fertility is not substantially altered by the computation of I_g', and the considerations of the preceding paragraph still remain basically valid. We will only remark that the corrected index of marital fertility shows a slower and later decline in the northern districts than appears from the uncorrected one; therefore the gap between north and south becomes more accentuated.

[8] The importance of the influence of emigration on fertility, because of the separation of husband and wife, was taken into consideration by Almeida Garrett, "Os problemas," *op. cit.*, *R.C.E.D.*, n.5, p. 97ff., who adopted a correction factor of fertility analogous to our own. See also Descamps, *op. cit.*, p. 70.

Table 19. Corrected Index of Marital Fertility (I'_g) by District

1890 - 1960

Districts	1890 (1888-92)	1900 (1901-04)	1911 (1909-13)	1920 (1918-22)	1930 (1928-32)	1940 (1938-42)	1950 (1948-52)	1960 (1958-62)
1. Bragança	.738	.693	.686	.816	.749	.602	.583	.507
2. Vila Real	.723	.691	.695	.750	.781	.582	.609	.607
3. Viana do Castelo	.772	.665	.734	.777	.767	.625	.648	.597
4. Braga	.774	.701	.688	.779	.759	.677	.774	.757
5. Porto	.697	.739	.689	.631	.597	.502	.555	.543
6. Guarda	.774	.796	.786	.752	.691	.595	.546	.480
7. Viseu	.783	.752	.726	.792	.684	.603	.588	.546
8. Aveiro	.792	.810	.772	.751	.690	.557	.552	.525
9. Castelo Branco	.735	.771	.729	.724	.628	.512	.445	.384
10. Coimbra	.713	.657	.638	.627	.531	.436	.419	.379
11. Leiria	.756	.694	.711	.653	.460	.496	.447	.386
12. Santarém	.691	.679	.605	.580	.491	.391	.353	.339
13. Lisbon	.552	.559	.540	.427	.332	.230	.236	.261
14. Portalegre	.666	.662	.642	.621	.520	.381	.316	.274
15. Évora	.610	.691	.625	.603	.501	.385	.320	.254
16. Setúbal	-	-	-	-	.445	.314	.245	.197
17. Beja	.639	.672	.640	.606	.542	.429	.375	.300
18. Faro	.702	.658	.646	.564	.448	.324	.295	.258
19. Angra	.733	.736	.746	.674	.568	.472	.488	.512
20. Horta	.690	.747	.684	.612	.507	.415	.392	.423
21. Ponta Delgada	.814	.871	.794	.753	.648	.570	.595	.677
22. Funchal	.816	.791	.811	.752	.775	.680	.711	.734
Portugal	.709	.700	.674	.642	.542	.468	.459	.435

Table 20. Index Numbers of (I'_g), 1890 = 100

Districts	1890	1900	1911	1920	1930	1940	1950	1960
1. Bragança	100	93.9	93.0	110.6	101.5	81.6	79.0	68.7
2. Vila Real	100	95.6	96.1	103.7	108.0	80.5	84.2	84.0
3. Viana do Castelo	100	86.1	95.1	100.6	99.4	81.0	83.9	77.3
4. Braga	100	90.6	88.9	100.6	98.1	87.5	100.0	97.8
5. Porto	100	106.0	98.9	90.5	85.7	72.0	79.6	77.9
6. Guarda	100	102.8	101.6	97.2	89.3	76.9	70.5	62.0
7. Viseu	100	96.0	92.7	101.1	87.4	77.0	75.1	69.7
8. Aveiro	100	102.3	97.5	94.8	87.1	70.3	69.7	66.3
9. Castelo Branco	100	104.9	99.2	98.5	85.4	69.7	60.5	52.2
10. Coimbra	100	92.1	89.5	87.9	74.5	61.1	58.8	53.2
11. Leiria	100	91.8	94.0	86.4	60.8	65.6	59.1	51.1
12. Santarém	100	98.3	87.6	83.9	71.1	56.6	51.1	49.1
13. Lisbon	100	101.3	97.8	77.4	60.1	41.7	42.8	47.3
14. Portalegre	100	99.3	96.4	93.2	78.1	57.2	47.4	41.4
15. Évora	100	113.2	102.5	98.9	82.1	63.1	52.5	41.6
16. Setúbal	-	-	-	-	-	-	-	-
17. Beja	100	105.2	100.2	94.8	84.8	67.1	58.7	46.9
18. Faro	100	93.7	92.0	80.3	63.8	46.2	42.0	36.8
19. Angra	100	100.4	101.8	92.0	77.5	64.4	66.6	69.9
20. Horta	100	108.3	99.1	88.7	73.5	60.1	56.8	61.3
21. Ponta Delgada	100	107.0	97.5	93.7	79.6	70.0	73.1	83.2
22. Funchal	100	96.9	99.4	93.4	95.0	83.3	87.1	90.0
Portugal	100	98.7	95.1	90.6	76.4	66.7	64.7	61.4

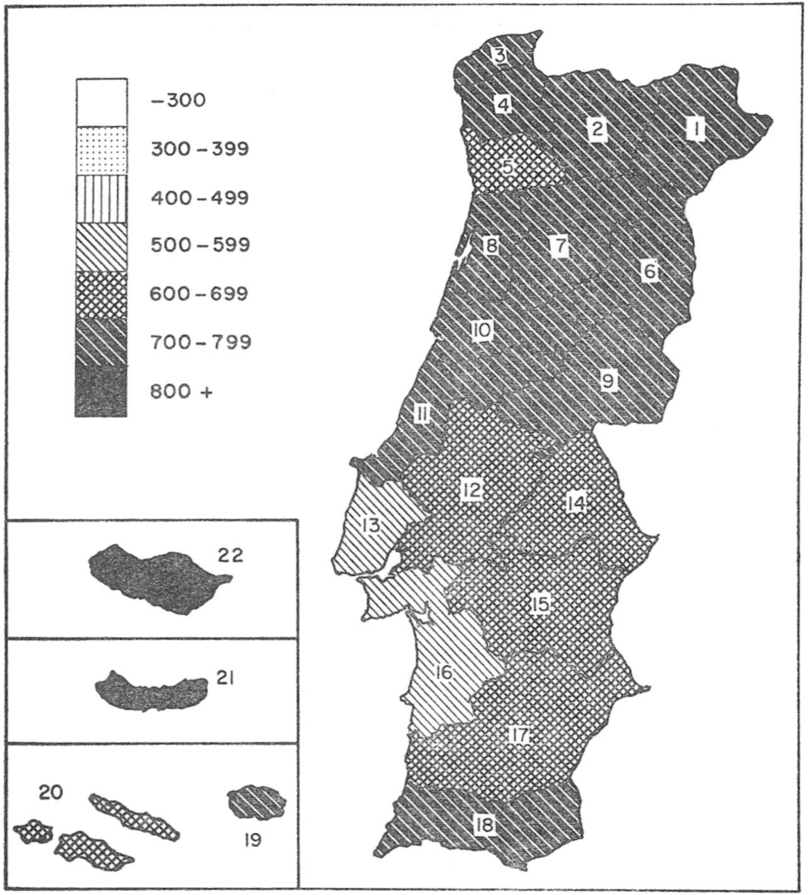

Figure 4a. Adjusted index of marital fertility, I_g', 1890

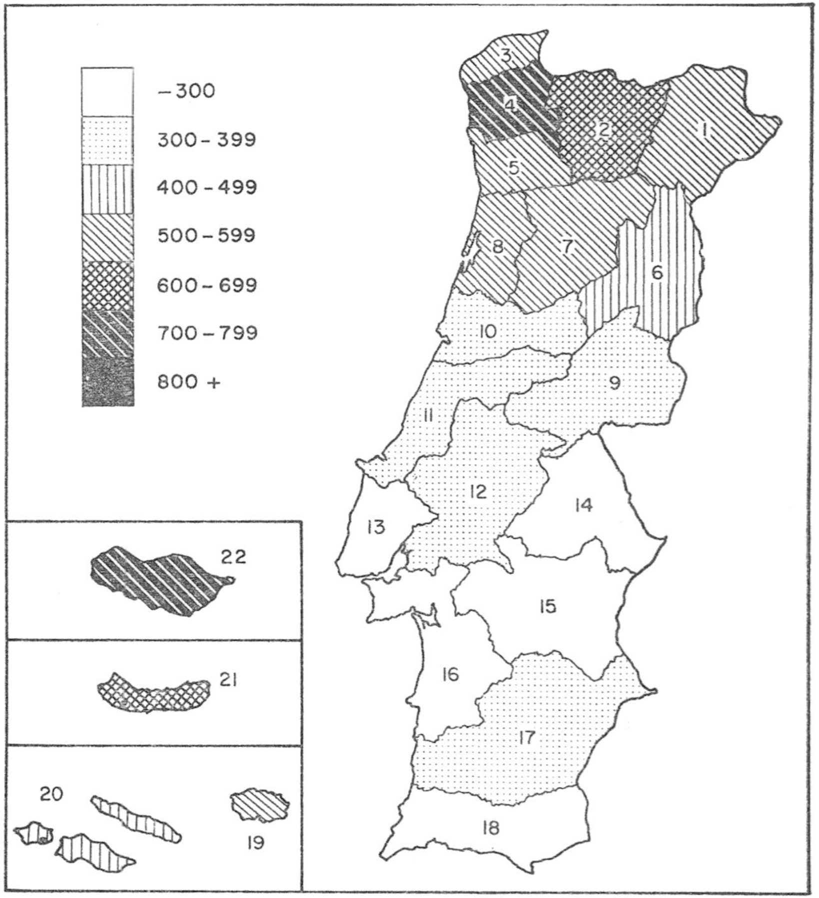

Figure 4b. Adjusted index of marital fertility, I_g', 1960

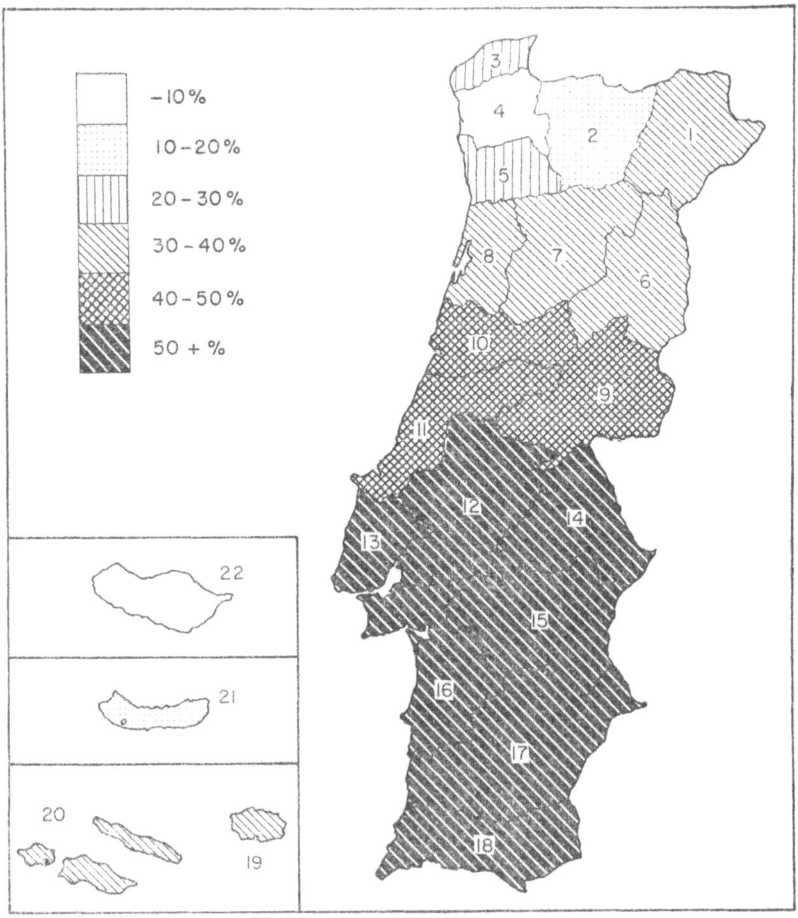

Figure 5. Percentage decrease in the adjusted index of marital fertility, I_g', 1890-1960

5.4. *Illegitimacy*

Illegitimacy, in Portugal, is among the highest in Europe, close to Austria and Sweden, contrasting with the low levels prevailing in other Latin countries. For the whole of Portugal illegitimacy remains almost constant until 1940 and rapidly decreases in the last two decades. A closer look at the annual series of data reveals, however, a strong surge of illegitimacy after the Concordat of 1928 and the change in the marriage legislation. The percent of total births that were illegitimate rose from 12 to nearly 16 in 1937;

from that date on there is a continuous decline (7.5 percent in 1966). The increase of illegitimacy after 1928 is shown also by the index of illegitimate fertility (.075 in 1920 and 1940, but .088 in 1930).

At the end of the last century, illegitimacy was rather high (I_h over .100) in certain districts of the north (Bragança, Vila Real, Viseu, Porto) and in Lisbon. Two factors are responsible for these high levels: the first is the disproportion of sexes caused by emigration; the second, low nuptiality, and particularly the high proportion of females remaining single. Since a large fraction of the female population was forcibly excluded from marriage, it is not surprising to find a high number of illegitimate conceptions, often tolerated by the family and the society. Descamps points out, talking about the Minho, "that married men and unmarried women enjoy ample freedom. This is because of the effects of the numerical disproportion of sexes and because of the mixing together, since the young ages, of boys and girls for work in the fields."[9] It is likely that the slow but steady increase of nuptiality was the main factor in the reduction of illegitimacy.

In the districts south of the Tagus, illegitimacy was for the most part above the national average, but this certainly cannot be imputed to emigration or nuptiality, the first almost nonexistent, the second around normal levels. But other conditions existed favoring illegitimacy in the south: on the one hand there was the relatively high frequency of "irregular" couples (already pointed out in 4.3), living "more uxorio," whose offspring were registered as illegitimate; and, on the other hand there was the high incidence of internal seasonal influx of male and female migrant workers who often lived in complete promiscuity in the large estates of Alentejo. Montalvão Machado observes that "in the *montes* (farms) of Alentejo, often 40 to 60 persons of different ages and sexes live promiscuously in the same room."[10]

The high illegitimacy of Lisbon can be explained by the con-

[9] Descamps, *op. cit.*, p. 84.
[10] Montalvão Machado, "Alguns," *op. cit.*, p. 135.

tinuous immigration of young women employed in domestic service and, generally speaking, by the poor social conditions prevailing there, as in many urban centers and seaports of Europe.

Finally, it has to be noted that many children registered as illegitimate were legitimated by the subsequent marriage of the irregular couple ("when they have two or three children they perform the civil marriage"). This sequence often occurred in the south (see Table 21), where the ratio of legitimated to illegitimate

Table 21. Births Legitimated through Marriage as Percent of Illegitimate Births

	1940	1950		1940	1950
Bragança	8.6	13.1	Santarém	10.4	17.4
Vila Real	3.8	9.9	Lisbon	12.3	15.8
Viana do Castelo	13.1	16.1	Portalegre	37.1	35.0
Braga	7.5	8.4	Évora	15.2	35.1
Porto	5.0	5.6	Setúbal	13.9	10.1
Guarda	7.2	15.6	Beja	2.5	5.6
Viseu	14.3	17.3	Faro	26.9	25.4
Aveiro	15.0	9.3	Angra	2.6	6.0
Castelo Branco	8.9	16.8	Horta	3.5	42.1
Coimbra	16.2	12.9	Ponta Delgada	25.3	7.4
Leiria	12.0	18.5	Funchal	8.5	5.5
			Portugal	11.8	14.0

births reached 1/4 to 1/3, in Portalegre, Évora, and Faro. Clearly enough, many births, formally illegitimate, were substantially legitimate, since they issued from parents who lived together but remained unmarried only because the ceremony was costly.[11]

Summing up the findings of this section, we may observe that:

(1) The changes in illegitimacy from the end of the nineteenth century to the present (Table 22) are probably related to the strong increase in nuptiality in the north, where the index of illegitimate

[11] Descamps, *op. cit.*, p. 85.

Table 22. Index of Illegitimate Fertility (I_h) by District

Districts	1890 (1888-92)	1900 (1901-04)	1911 (1909-13)	1920 (1918-22)	1930 (1928-32)	1940 (1938-42)	1950 (1948-52)	1950 (1958-62)
1. Braganca	.137	.113	.114	.114	.104	.108	-	.112
2. Vila Real	.126	.108	.101	.111	.129	-	.091	.072
3. Viana do Castelo	.050	.059	.062	.063	.070	.058	.051	.034
4. Braga	.059	.055	.054	.056	.061	.053	.046	.032
5. Porto	.092	.087	.094	.074	.088	.072	.063	.058
6. Guarda	.068	.049	.047	.039	.048	.034	.024	.015
7. Viseu	.100	.080	.082	.078	.078	.070	.056	.040
8. Aveiro	.057	.058	.056	.055	.057	.054	.044	.039
9. Castelo Branco	.040	.033	.027	.028	.027	.024	.018	.014
10. Coimbra	.049	.036	.046	.040	.039	.035	.031	.029
11. Leiria	.040	.044	.049	.053	.075	.075	.058	.046
12. Santarém	.048	.063	.053	.047	.063	.061	-	.050
13. Lisbon	.108	.135	.165	.132	.124	.091	.069	.076
14. Portalegre	.060	.061	.062	.060	.065	.076	.057	.058
15. Évora	.080	.093	.112	.112	.134	.136	.100	.085
16. Setúbal	-	-	-	-	.221	.189	.142	.121
17. Beja	.080	.081	.092	.098	.100	.110	.114	.114
18. Faro	.068	.076	.093	.087	.097	.113	.093	.072
19. Angra	.058	.041	.018	.024	.020	.021	.023	.028
20. Horta	.043	.033	.027	.022	.027	.031	.027	.017
21. Ponta Delgada	.023	.014	.013	.008	.011	.018	.010	.010
22. Funchal	.033	.018	.014	.013	.015	.017	.018	.015
Portugal	.075	.073	.083	.075	.088	.076	.059	.057

fertility had decreased, and to the stagnation of nuptiality in the south, where illegitimacy has shown little change.

(2) The findings in (1) can be confirmed by the correlation—in the expected sense—existing between changes in nuptiality and changes in illegitimacy from 1890 to 1960:

r (percent of changes of I_m and I_h, 1890-1960)	$= -.475$
r (percent of changes in the proportion of females remaining single, age 50-54, and of I_h, 1890-1960)	$= +.716$

(3) The impact of illegitimacy on total fertility $[I_h \, . \, (1 - I_m)/I_f]$ is often high, between 10 and 13 percent for the whole country, but reaching 1/3 in Setúbal (1930) and 1/4 in Évora, Vila Real (1930), and Lisbon. Finally, part of the variations of illegitimacy are "apparent" and derive from the changes in the marriage legislation of 1911 and 1928.

5.5. *Other Aspects of Fertility Trends*

A few additional elaborations may be useful for a better appraisal of Portuguese fertility. We have thought it useful, in the first place, to compute the values of the territorial variability of the various indices of nuptiality and fertility (I_m, I_f, I_g, I_g'), from 1890 to 1960; the results (sigma and cv) are reported in Table 23. The coefficient of variability (cv) of the proportion married (I_m) tends to decrease, while the variability of fertility tends to increase. The increase of cv, between 1890 and 1960, is larger for marital fertility (4 times for I_g; 3.7 for I_g') than for general fertility (I_f). There is an obvious compensating influence of nuptiality (I_m) which, increasing more in the north than in the south, has partially balanced the decline of marital fertility, larger in the north than in the south.

One of the principal aims of this study is to determine the approximate date of the start of fertility decline. Assuming the two criteria already described (see 4.1.), we may construct Table 24:

Table 23. Territorial Variability of Nuptiality and Fertility, 1890-1960

Year	Sigma	Mean	cv	cv index n. (1890=100)	Sigma	Mean	cv	cv index n. (1890=100)
	Index of the proportion married (I_m)				Index of general fertility (I_f)			
1890	57.66	.458	12.59	100	42.09	.359	11.72	100
1900	57.18	.465	12.30	98	46.78	.361	12.96	111
1911	56.67	.488	11.61	92	43.05	.355	12.13	103
1920	56.75	.468	12.13	96	41.72	.334	12.49	107
1930	46.48	.486	9.56	76	45.08	.317	14.22	121
1940	52.08	.490	10.63	84	47.27	.271	17.44	149
1950	45.73	.499	9.16	73	58.05	.264	21.99	188
1960	50.24	.557	9.02	72	71.45	.261	27.38	234
	Index of marital fertility (I_g)				Corrected index of marital fertility (I'_g)			
1890	60.03	.698	8.60	100	67.12	.718	9.35	100
1900	66.08	.696	9.49	110	60.32	.716	8.42	90
1910	58.42	.656	8.91	104	62.61	.695	11.10	119
1920	83.72	.644	13.00	151	104.56	.679	15.40	165
1930	116.65	.598	19.51	227	134.00	.596	22.48	240
1940	129.67	.482	26.90	313	147.20	.498	29.56	316
1950	136.01	.457	29.76	346	152.77	.477	32.03	342
1960	146.80	.430	34.14	397	154.96	.452	34.28	367

The two methods give rather different results; the second of the two seems to be more gradual and, on the whole, more consistent, setting an arbitrary but precise borderline between "high" and weakly controlled, and "low" but more efficiently controlled, fertility. The second method establishes a clear distinction between the districts of the south, all included in the upper section of our table, and the districts of the north, which only in recent years approach relatively low levels of fertility.

The analysis of territorial trends of fertility suggests some further reflections. We have spoken, in the preceding pages, of the strong

Table 24. Date of Decline of Marital Fertility

	Marital fertility (I_g) falls:	
	10% below the 1890 level	below .600
before 1890	--	Lisbon
1890 - 1900	--	--
1900 - 1910	Coimbra, Santarém	--
1911 - 1920	Leiria, Lisbon, Faro, Horta	Santarém, Faro
1920 - 1930	Porto, Guarda, Aveiro, Castelo Branco, Évora, Beja, Angra, Ponta Delgada	Porto, Coimbra, Leiria, Portalegre, Évora, Beja, Angra, Horta
1930 - 1940	Bragança, Vila Real, Viana do Castelo, Funchal, Portalegre	Guarda, Aveira, Castelo Branco, Ponta Delgada
1940 - 1950	--	Bragança, Viseu
1950 - 1960	--	Viana do Castelo
after 1960	Braga	Vila Real, Braga, Funchal

contrast between the north and the south; we shall add now that the islands have, on the average, a marital fertility higher than the north, while the center area of transition is closer to the south than to the north. However, the influence of the low fertility and early decline of Lisbon and Coimbra makes the center a peculiar case, of little use for our argument. The north and the islands are slow in adopting neomalthusian techniques and principles of fertility control, while in the south these techniques were widely and rapidly accepted. We will discuss in Chapter 7 the factors that may have influenced this differential evolution, but we would like to point out here a different aspect of the problem. Before the beginning of the fertility decline, there were substantial differences between the levels of fertility of the various areas, as can be seen in the table below, where the mean values of I_g and I_g' for the north, the center, the south, and the islands have been reported:

Area	Index of marital fertility, (I_g)			Corrected index of marital fertility, (I'_g)		
	1890	1900	1911	1890	1900	1911
North	.723	.699	.660	.752	.731	.722
Center	.677	.652	.615	.689	.672	.645
South	.650	.669	.628	.654	.671	.638
Islands	.739	.773	.725	.763	.786	.759
North/South	1.112	1.045	1.051	1.157	1.089	1.132
Highest/Lowest	1.137	1.186	1.179	1.167	1.171	1.190

There is no doubt that substantial differences between the north (and the islands) and the south exist at all three dates retained here. The differences are not large for I_g in 1900 and 1911, but this may be explained by the depressive influence on marital fertility determined by the rising mass emigration from the district of the north, starting at the end of the century. Let us compare the levels of I_g', where the effects of emigration are eliminated (although not completely). The differences in fertility (I_g') between the north and the south are indeed notable, varying between 9 and 16 percent; the differences between the area with highest (islands) and the area with lowest fertility (south) are even larger, around 17-19 percent.

One implication of these "pre-decline" differences in marital fertility may be the possible compensating influence of the propensity to marriage, much higher in the south than in the north. The population of the north, more fertile because of natural, biological, or social factors, would resort to more extreme checks of the malthusian type, such as postponement or avoidance of marriage, in order to limit the frequency of births. On the other hand, the population of the south, less pressed by the problems of a high fertility, would feel less need to limit marriages.

Still, the factors underlying the different fertility levels of the north and the south, before the onset of the secular decline, remain unexplained. It is not possible to evaluate the influence of morbid or biological factors in determining the relatively low fertility of the south; but we may exclude the existence of differences in sterility, as we will clearly see further on.

Descamps observed that in the Minho children were weaned when they were only a few months old, and this could account both for the higher infant mortality of the region and for a hypothetical lower mean birth interval corresponding to a higher fertility. But except for the observation of Descamps which, on the other hand, is contradicted by other sources (see Conclusion), we have been unable to find support for this hypothesis.

We are of the opinion that the voluntary control of fertility cannot be ruled out as a factor contributing to the fertility gap even before the modern sustained decline began. It is possible that the southern population had already to some extent begun to practice efficient, even if primitive, techniques of fertility control at the end of the last century.

CHAPTER 6: Fertility, Family Size, and Sterility

6.1. *Family Size and Sterility According to the 1940 Census*

The censuses of 1940, 1950, and 1960 asked married women a few questions about the number of children ever born to them. These data, adequately elaborated, offer valuable information not otherwise available. First of all, the censuses make it possible to know the completed size of Portuguese families, a useful measure in itself of fertility, and also important because of its presumed effect on the motivation to control fertility. It is also possible to measure the level of sterility of the married women, an important element for the knowledge of a relevant biological aspect of fertility. Secondarily, census statistics make it possible to measure the fertility of different cohorts, and, therefore, the timing of the decline. Finally, census cohort data, if compared with the period measures presented in the preceding chapter, provide a control of consistency between the two types of fertility measures.

Table 25 contains the data for 1940 on the average number of children ever born to married females 40-44 years old and 45 years old and over, who had been married for at least twenty years.[1] In the same table, the proportion of sterile women is reported. It has to be pointed out that the levels of fertility and sterility for the two groups of women (40-44 and 45 and over) cannot be compared. This is because the married women of 40-44 years had all been married before the age of 25, while the married women over 45 (whose marriages had a duration of at least 20 years) could have married also at relatively older ages, thus decreasing the average fertility level of the group (and increasing

[1] The 1940 census reports the distribution of married women according to the following classes of children ever born: 1-2, 3-4, 5-7, 8-10, 11-13, 14-16, 17, and over. The total number of children ever born has been computed applying to the above reported distribution the following weights: 1.6, 3.6, 6.0, 8.7, 11.7, 14.5, and 17.5. The weights have been computed on the basis of the complete distribution of married females by number of living children, reported in the same census volume.

Table 25. Average Number of Children Ever Born to Women Married 20 Years or More and Percent of Women Without Children, by District, 1940 Census

Districts	Females married 20 or more years			
	children ever born		percent without children	
	40-44 (1)	45+ (2)	40-44 (3)	45+ (4)
1. Bragança	6.87	6.09	4.0	6.3
2. Vila Real	6.60	6.06	3.3	6.0
3. Viana do Castelo	5.78	5.49	2.4	6.6
4. Braga	7.13	6.20	2.7	5.4
5. Porto	5.56	6.05	5.3	7.1
6. Guarda	6.19	5.76	2.9	5.6
7. Viseu	5.93	5.55	3.3	5.4
8. Aveiro	5.66	5.44	3.6	6.2
9. Castelo Branco	5.67	3.60	2.4	5.4
10. Coimbra	4.57	4.42	3.6	6.2
11. Leiria	5.29	4.88	4.5	7.0
12. Santarém	4.51	4.65	4.3	5.5
13. Lisbon	3.71	3.75	9.4	13.6
14. Portalegre	4.86	5.04	4.9	6.0
15. Évora	5.26	5.08	5.3	7.7
16. Setúbal	5.00	5.06	4.8	7.7
17. Beja	5.66	5.10	8.6	6.2
18. Faro	4.21	4.59	3.6	6.2
19. Angra	5.81	6.12	3.6	6.0
20. Horta	5.37	5.52	3.7	6.2
21. Ponta Delgada	6.97	6.61	2.8	5.2
22. Funchal	7.16	6.86	3.3	4.3
Portugal	5.32	5.23	4.7	7.1

its sterility). Moreover, it should be noted that, especially in illiterate populations, there is a widespread tendency for older women to understate their parity.

It is clear that the first of the two groups is "selected" for an early age at marriage, which, on the average, must have been around 20 years. It is easy to explain, therefore, why the older women have in many instances (see Table 25) a lower average number children and a higher sterility than the younger age group.

The data on Table 25 show, for the two groups of females considered, an average number of children around 5.2-5.3. The data indicate a level of fertility not exceptionally high, and slightly below the fertility of Italian married women shown in the 1931 census.[2] Territorial variability is very high; the average number of children per married woman of 40-44 years of age runs from a minimum of 3.7 for the district of Lisbon to a maximum of 7.1-7.2 for Braga and Madeira. The spatial variation is shown in Figure 6.

It is encouraging to note the close relationship between the average number of children per married woman, resulting from the census data, and the index of marital fertility (I_g) in the various districts. The average number of children per woman 40 to 44 years of age has been correlated with the average of I_g in 1920 and 1930; it is in that period that the women who were 40-44 in 1940 experienced their highest fertility (between 1920 and 1930, their ages were between 20 and 34 years). The family size of the older age group of 45 years and over has been related to the indices of marital fertility computed for 1911 and for 1920; however, this being an open age group, its relationship with a current measure of fertility such as I_g is rather imprecise.

The results of the correlation analysis are the following:

r, I_g 1920-30 and average number of children ever had by married women of 40-44 years (1940) $= +.934$

r, I_g 1911, and average number of children ever had by married women of 45 years and over (1940) $= +.830$

r, I_g 1920 and average number of children ever had by married women of 45 years and over (1940) $= +.851$

The high correlation found between measures of fertility drawn from the census, on the one hand, and from the current statistics, on the other, attests to the reliability and adequacy of the standard-

[2] In the 1931 census, the average number of children ever born per Italian married woman (all ages at marriage) over the age of 45 was 5.45.

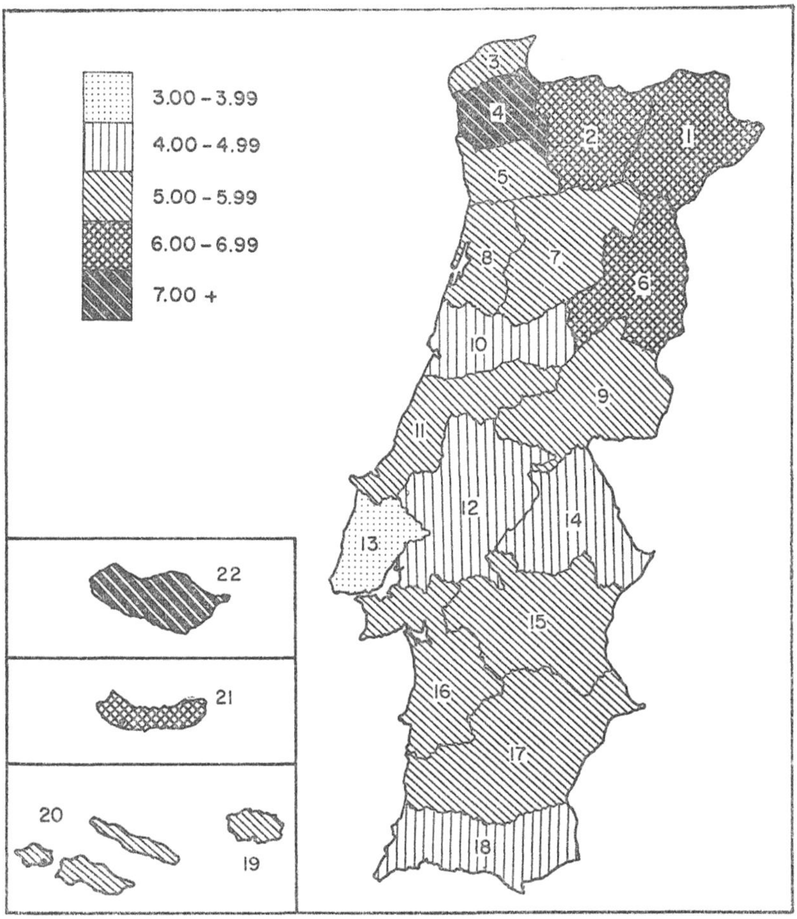

Figure 6. Average number of children ever born to married women 40-44 years, married 20 years or more, 1940

ized index of marital fertility in illustrating fertility trends and differentials.

There is yet another consideration which seems of some interest. Let us assume that the average age of the married women 40 to 44 years was 42.5 years. We know that they had been married for at least 20 years and as many as 30 years (supposing 15 years the minimum age at marriage). If we set the average duration of marriage at 22.5 years we will not be far from the truth. In other words, this means that the average age at marriage for this group of women was 20 years. Now, the average number of children ever born to a Hutterite female (married at the age of 20) by the age of 42.5 years, would be equal to

$$D = \sum_{20}^{42.5} f_x^H = 10.2$$

where f_x^H are the age specific legitimate fertility rates of the Hutterite women (marriages of 1921-1930), and the standard fertility schedule adopted for the various indices of fertility adopted in this study. If we divide the average number of children ever born to the 40-44 married women (according to the census) by 10.2, we obtain, in another way, an estimate of I_g, which can compare with the average I_g (computed on the basis of the current statistics) for 1920-1930. The comparison between the two series of values can be done in Table 26. The two estimates of I_g are very close, although they cannot coincide for obvious reasons: Generally it is the I_g computed from the census data which is slightly lower, as is to be expected, since women, 40-44 and married 20 years, are probably concentrated to some extent toward the upper end of the age range, had been married somewhat less than 22.5 years, and were married at an average age somewhat above 20.

The data on average family size lend themselves to further comment. Marital fertility of the four provinces north of the Douro river (Bragança, Vila Real, Viana do Castelo, and Braga) showed no tendency to decline until 1930 or thereabout. The persistence in that area of high values of legitimate fertility may be attributed to the lack of voluntary control of fertility prevailing in the population, a condition that can be thought of as living in a régime of "natural" fertility, to use Henry's terminology (see, however, the following section 6.4). The average number of children of the women 40 to 44 and married 20 years was, in that area, around 6.5, which compares with over 10 children of the Hutterite women; the mean interval between births—assuming that the first birth would take place when the mother was 21, and the last when she was 39 or 40 years old—was 3.3-3.5 years. Thus the level of fertility must be regarded as relatively low, and the interbirth inter-

Table 26. Index of Marital Fertility (I_g) Calculated and Estimated from the Census Fertility Data

Districts	Children ever born to married females 40 to 44, 20 years or more of marriage	Column (1) ÷ 10.2	Index of marital fertility (I_g), average 1920–30	Percent of difference between (2) & (3)
	(1)	(2)	(3)	(4)
1. Bragança	6.87	.674	.765	+13.5
2. Vila Real	6.60	.647	.733	+17.5
3. Viana do Castelo	5.78	.567	.678	+19.6
4. Braga	7.13	.699	.722	+ 3.3
5. Porto	5.56	.545	.581	+ 6.6
6. Guarda	6.19	.607	.674	+11.0
7. Viseu	5.93	.581	.659	+13.4
8. Aveiro	5.66	.555	.638	+15.0
9. Castelo Branco	5.67	.556	.661	+18.8
10. Coimbra	4.57	.448	.523	+16.7
11. Leiria	5.29	.519	.529	+ 1.9
12. Santarém	4.51	.442	.529	+19.7
13. Lisbon	3.71	.364	.380	+ 4.4
14. Portalegre	4.86	.476	.564	+18.5
15. Évora	5.26	.516	.548	+ 6.2
16. Setúbal	5.00	.490	.500	+ 2.0
17. Beja	5.66	.555	.572	+ 3.1
18. Faro	4.21	.413	.482	+16.7
19. Angra	5.81	.570	.611	+ 7.2
20. Horta	5.37	.526	.550	+ 4.6
21. Ponta Delgada	6.97	.683	.680	− 0.4
22. Funchal	7.13	.702	.740	+ 5.4
Portugal	5.32	.522	.576	+10.3

vals as relatively long. The possible action of biological factors has to be ruled out, since the level of sterility in the group did not exceed 3 percent, a level even lower than that of the Hutterites. Emigration could be regarded as a factor in determining the relatively low level of marital fertility. The temporary or permanent emigration of the husband certainly causes—other factors remaining equal—a lower level of fertility of the wife. On the other hand, emigration is certainly a selective process, not only with regard to sex, age, and marital status, but also from the social, psychological, and even biological point of view. When emigration is permanent, and when the mechanism of selection stimulates the departure of the more active and open minded section of the population, emigration can be regarded as a factor of conservation of the existing social structure, probably opposing the process of diffusion of a control-minded attitude of the population. Given the scarce elements at our disposal, a careful appraisal of the nature of Portuguese emigration becomes difficult, and it is impossible to assess its role and impact on fertility, which certainly is not of a simple nature.

It is therefore our opinion that the gap between "standard" fertility—the fertility of the Hutterites or of any other group with high levels of natural fertility—and the fertility of the provinces of the north can be ascribed neither to the level of sterility nor to the high rate of emigration, whose effects on fertility are, at least, controversial.

In all of Portugal, the sterility of women 40 to 44 and married 20 years or more is very low, with the exception of Lisbon and Beja, where approximately 9 percent of women are sterile.[3] In the other districts, sterility never exceeds 5 percent, and in 14 out of 22 districts sterility lies between 3 and 4 percent. Moreover, a significant negative correlation is found between sterility and the

[3] It would be more correct to talk about "childlessness," instead of sterility, which implies a medical-physiological notion. As to the level of sterility, it is important to report the following considerations drawn from Whelpton, Campbell, and Patterson, *Fertility and Family Planning in the United States*, Princeton, 1966, p. 163: "Extremely low proportions with no children have been reported for certain population groups. For example, Tietze found only 2.4 percent childless among 209 Hutterite women who had married before age 25, had spent 20 years or more with the same husband, and had not used contraception. Among ever-married women 30 to 44 years old living in rural farm areas of Utah, the proportion childless is only 3.1 percent, according to the 1960 Census. Proportions between 3 and 5 percent are shown by the 1910 Census for ever-married women over 40 who were born in Russia or Poland."

average number of children per married woman 40 to 44 (—.693). It is evident that while biological sterility was probably around 2 or 3 percent in all districts, the diffusion of neomalthusian techniques has caused an increase in the proportion of women remaining voluntarily sterile in the provinces where marital fertility was lowest. Finally, sterility in the married woman over 45 years of age is higher than in the younger generation. This is no surprise, because in this group are included those women who married at an advanced age, and were therefore sterile since the beginning of marriage.

In Table 27 we have reported the proportion of sterile married women in each age group (all durations of marriage), for the provinces with the highest (Tras-os-Montes) and with the lowest (Estremadura) fertility, compared with the total Portuguese population. The differences are indeed striking; above age 25 sterility in Estremadura is two to three times higher than in Tras-os-Montes. The contrast reveals large differentials in the behavior of the couples; a sterility level between 15 and 20 percent (Estremadura) can be found only in populations where family limitation is almost universally adopted, while a sterility level of 6 to 7 percent (Tras-

Table 27. Proportion of Married Females Without Children, by Age, 1940 Census

				as percent of Portugal	
Age	Portugal	Tras-os-Montes	Estremadura	Tras-os-Montes	Estremadura
– 20	49.8	49.9	50.1	100.2	100.6
20-24	26.2	19.2	33.8	73.3	129.0
25-29	14.3	9.4	23.6	65.7	165.0
30-34	10.0	6.5	18.4	65.0	184.0
35-39	8.3	5.8	14.4	69.9	173.5
40-44	9.0	6.7	16.5	74.4	183.3
45 +	10.7	9.6	18.3	89.7	171.0
Total	11.9	9.3	19.6	78.2	164.7

os-Montes) is probably only slightly above the minimum, biological level.[4]

6.2. *The Fertility Surveys of 1950 and 1960*

The 1950 fertility survey is another important source of information for the study of fertility. Unfortunately, although data on births according to age of the mother and duration of marriage were collected, they cannot be exploited for our purposes. We will limit our analysis, therefore, to Table 28, where the average number of children ever born per ever-married woman is reported, by district, for different birth cohorts. The data of this table are not homogeneous with those of Table 25 because: a) the average number of children refers to ever-married women including widows, divorcées, etc., while in 1940 only the currently married women had been considered; b) no distinction by age at marriage or duration of marriage is made, and the average number of children refers to women having different lengths of married life.

Finally, in many instances, we will see that the mean number of children per woman increases passing from one cohort to the following, younger one (when fertility is falling, the contrary should be expected). This may be the effect a) of the selective action of mortality, eliminating at a faster rate the more fecund women, who belong also to the less favored social classes or b) to the under-reporting of events by the older women.

The evidence collected in Table 28 reveals a decline of the family size from 4.5 children per ever-married woman with completed fertility, and born before 1885, to about 4 for those born at the turn of the century (1895-1905). Once again the territorial detail confirms what has been often observed: the family size is stable (comparing the cohort born before 1875 and 1885 with that born in 1895-1905) in many districts of the north (Bragança, Vila Real, Braga), while the largest decline occurred in the center and in the south (Lisbon, Faro, Setúbal, Portalegre). The gap be-

[4] Again, the reader must be reminded that these values cannot be compared with those derived from Table 28.

Table 28. Average Number of Children Ever Born per Ever-Married Woman, 1950 Census

Districts	Year of Birth				Year of Birth			
	-1875	1875-1885	1885-1895	1895-1905	-1875	1875-1885	1885-1895	1895-1905
	Absolute values				Index numbers, 1875-1885=100			
1. Bragança	5.09	5.26	5.45	5.37	96.8	100	103.6	102.1
2. Vila Real	5.11	5.16	5.28	5.19	99.0	100	102.3	100.6
3. Viana do Castelo	4.54	4.58	4.56	4.28	99.1	100	99.6	93.4
4. Braga	4.93	5.05	5.19	5.08	97.6	100	102.8	100.6
5. Porto	4.91	4.74	4.49	4.06	103.6	100	94.7	85.7
6. Guarda	5.38	5.19	5.28	4.79	103.7	100	97.9	97.3
7. Viseu	4.69	4.64	4.72	4.38	101.1	100	101.7	94.4
8. Aveiro	4.57	4.60	4.53	4.00	94.3	100	98.5	87.0
9. Castelo Branco	4.98	5.00	4.76	4.48	99.6	100	95.2	89.6
10. Coimbra	3.92	3.88	3.78	3.41	101.0	100	97.4	87.9
11. Leiria	4.11	4.16	4.24	3.87	98.8	100	101.9	93.0
12. Santarém	4.12	4.12	4.01	3.58	100.0	100	97.3	89.3
13. Lisbon	3.82	3.44	3.04	2.61	111.0	100	98.4	75.9
14. Portalegre	4.69	4.72	4.51	3.96	99.4	100	95.6	83.9
15. Évora	4.44	4.40	4.52	4.18	100.9	100	102.7	95.0
16. Setúbal	4.59	4.57	4.33	3.68	100.4	100	94.7	80.5
17. Beja	4.41	4.63	4.66	4.35	95.2	100	100.6	94.0
18. Faro	4.41	4.02	3.90	3.38	109.7	100	97.0	84.1
19. Angra	4.74	5.05	5.05	4.34	93.9	100	100.0	85.9
20. Horta	4.17	4.80	4.61	3.89	86.8	100	96.0	81.0
21. Ponta Delgada	5.26	5.70	5.90	5.45	92.3	100	103.5	95.6
22. Funchal	5.43	5.53	5.86	5.48	98.2	100	106.0	99.1
Portugal	4.51	4.47	4.36	3.98	100.9	100	97.5	89.0

tween the north and the other areas of the continent is already evident for the women born before 1885 and, of course, it increases for the younger ones. The family size of women born before 1885 is 5 to 5.5 children in Bragança, Vila Real, Guarda, Braga, and Castelo Branco; below 4 in Coimbra and Lisbon; and between 4 and 4.5 in Leiria, Santarém, Faro, Beja, and Évora. The cohorts born before 1875 had probably almost completed their family size by 1910, and those born before 1885, by 1920; approximately the same territorial differentials are shown by the computation of the period fertility measures (I_g, I_g') computed before 1920, and already discussed in Chapter 5.

Let us make now a final check of consistency between the cohort and period fertility measures. We have supposed that the cohort born before 1875 had experienced its higher fertility around 1900; the 1875-1885 cohort, around 1911 and so on. The correlation coefficients between the two sets of measures run as follows:

1875 (and before) cohort and I_g of 1900	+.723
1875-1885 cohort and I_g of 1911	+.860
1885-1895 cohort and I_g of 1920	+.904
1895-1905 cohort and I_g of 1930	+.903

Taking into account the many factors that render very rough the correspondence between the two sets of measures, the results are encouraging, confirming the remarkable consistency between cohort and period measures.

The 1960 enumeration offers data on the number of children ever born to the married women, classified by age at census and age at marriage. These data are homogeneous with those derived from the 1940 census; unfortunately they have been tabulated for the whole Portuguese population, without territorial details (see Table 29). As was to be expected, the family size for women with the same age varies according to the age at marriage; those above 50 years of age had 4.9 children if married before the age of 20, but only 3.7 children if married between the ages of 25 and 30. The corresponding values, for women of 40 to 44 years, are 4.3 and 3.1. The completed family size (all durations of marriage) is

Table 29. Average Number of Children Ever Born per Married Woman, Portugal, 1960 Census

age at marriage \ age at census	– 20	20-24	25-29	30-34	35-39	40-44	45-49	50+	Total
– 20	.59	1.54	2.45	3.16	3.75	4.28	4.60	4.94	3.34
20-24		.81	1.68	2.56	3.20	3.74	3.99	4.35	3.06
25-29			.90	1.82	2.53	3.06	3.35	3.75	2.79
30-34				1.14	1.85	2.44	2.68	3.08	2.52
35-39					1.38	1.88	2.06	2.44	2.17
40-44						1.56	1.70	1.93	1.84
45-49							1.67	1.80	1.78
50+								2.02	2.02
Total	.59	1.14	1.67	2.37	2.94	3.39	3.59	3.84	2.94

3.84 for the women above age 50, and will be around 3.5 for those aged 35 to 44 who still had, in 1960, a short fecund life span before them.

If we compare the family size of the married women aged 40 to 44 in 1940 with a duration of marriage above 20 years, with the family size of the women having the same age and approximately the same duration of marriage in 1960, we come out with 5.32 children for the former against about 4.0 for the latter group. The conspicuous reduction of fertility between the two cohorts is evident.

Another hint as to the modifications of the reproductive behavior of the population can be derived from Table 30, where we have reported the proportion of sterile women by age, 1940 and 1960 censuses. The increase of sterility is substantial in each age group, and indicates the rapid diffusion of neomalthusian principles and practices throughout the population.

6.3. *Marital Fertility by Age, 1930-1960*

Starting in 1930, Portuguese vital statistics report births according to their legitimacy and the age of the mother. It is possible,

Table 30. Proportion Without Children, Ever-married Women, by Age (Portugal)

Age	1940	1960	1960 as percent of 1940
– 20	49.8	54.9	110.2
20-24	26.2	30.9	117.9
25-29	14.3	16.6	116.1
30-34	10.0	10.8	108.0
35-39	8.3	9.7	116.9
40-44	9.0	10.8	120.0
45+	10.7	14.4	134.6
Total	11.9	14.7	123.5

therefore, to compute age-specific marital fertility rates (from now on referred to as ASMFR) in correspondence with the four last censuses, and for the various districts.[5] It is true that the extensive material already examined is sufficient for a detailed appraisal of fertility trends, but the study of ASMFR may reveal, beside the notions already known, further aspects of the fertility decline which it is necessary to discuss.

In Table 31 we report, for the whole Portuguese population, the ASMFR, 1930-1960, and the corresponding index numbers, 1930 = 100. There is an evident differential pattern of decline of fertility according to the age of the mother; the percent decline of ASMFR increases going from the young to the older age groups (−8 percent for the 15-19 age group; −68 percent for the 45-49 age group, from 1930 to 1960). All that is, of course, well in line with the developments of fertility in other populations: in the phase of the decline, there is a tendency for fertility to concentrate in the

[5] The computation of ASMFR by district has required some elaboration of the data. For 1930, the distribution by age of illegitimate births was unknown. For each district we have proceeded to the distribution of total illegitimate births by age applying the percentage distribution of the illegitimate births of 1940 (total Portugal). In 1950, legitimate births by age included stillbirths. For each district the ratio, total live legitimate births/total legitimate births, has been computed and applied to each age group for the estimate of the number of legitimate live births.

Table 31. Age Specific Marital Fertility Rates for Portugal, 1930-1960

Ages	Age specific legitimate fertility rates				Index number, 1930=100			
	1930	1940	1950	1960	1930	1940	1950	1960
15-19	451.9	397.8	395.7	415.0	100	88.0	87.6	91.8
20-24	398.3	327.4	339.2	350.8	100	82.2	85.2	88.1
25-29	291.3	251.8	239.8	245.6	100	86.4	82.3	84.3
30-34	222.0	185.2	172.6	160.2	100	83.4	77.7	72.2
35-39	176.3	137.6	128.5	111.9	100	78.0	72.9	63.5
40-44	84.5	69.2	60.7	51.2	100	81.9	71.8	60.6
45-49	15.5	9.9	9.2	5.0	100	63.8	59.4	32.3

young ages, when procreation is less burdensome from both a psychological and physiological point of view.

Table 32 reports the marital fertility rates for the district with highest (and constant through time) fertility (Braga) and for the district with the lowest fertility (Faro). The contrast between the two districts, at the opposite ends of Portugal, and far apart in socioeconomic characteristics, is indeed striking. In Braga, fertility remains almost constant in almost all age groups between 1930 and 1960; in Faro, the percent decline ranges from slightly below 1/4 to almost 3/4. The fertility of Faro was, on the average, 1/2 the fertility of Braga in 1930 and only 1/3 or less in 1960.

Our data suggest further points of interest. In 1930, for instance, the fertility of at least three districts of the continent had remained unchanged since the end of the nineteenth century: Bragança ($I_g = .749$ in 1930 against .738 in 1890), Vila Real (.758 against .714), and Braga (.730 against .749). It is not hazardous to say that in these districts fertility was still in its premodern, predecline stage still untouched by the process of diffusion of neomalthusian ideas and practices. Still, fertility in this area is only 3/4 of the fertility of the Hutterites, and it is likely that it has never in the past surpassed this ratio.

There are two possible interpretations of this fact. With the first interpretation one could explain the constant level of fertility by assuming that no control whatsoever is exercised on fertility, which

Table 32. Age Specific Marital Fertility Rates in Braga and Faro

Age	1930	1940	1950	1960	Percent of change, 1960/1930
			Braga		
20-24	470.2	363.9	465.0	493.5	+ 5.0
25-29	385.3	345.7	375.4	398.3	+ 3.4
30-34	315.6	316.3	303.6	291.2	− 7.7
35-39	255.7	234.6	238.3	232.4	− 9.1
40-44	114.6	113.7	123.9	110.6	− 3.5
45-49	18.7	15.4	18.0	11.6	−38.0
			Faro		
20-24	317.1	264.2	248.0	245.4	−22.6
25-29	214.0	175.6	144.1	140.7	−34.3
30-34	151.6	121.9	92.6	77.1	−49.1
35-39	115.3	87.7	67.1	44.2	−61.7
40-44	45.4	33.7	25.3	18.9	−58.4
45-49	9.3	6.0	3.1	2.5	−73.1
			Faro as percent of Braga		
20-24	67.4	72.6	53.3	49.8	-
25-29	55.5	50.8	38.4	35.3	-
30-34	48.0	38.5	30.5	26.5	-
35-39	45.1	37.4	28.2	19.0	-
40-44	39.6	29.6	20.4	17.1	-
45-49	49.7	39.0	17.2	21.6	-

is determined only by natural factors (sterility, length of breast-feeding, etc.). With the second interpretation one could say that the level of fertility, lower than the empirical maximum, is imputable to voluntary control which, because of the relatively rigid social structure and lack of territorial, social, and cultural mobility, remained limited to certain segments of the population, or to certain age groups or periods of life, without further extensions. If the first interpretation is true, the decline of fertility from one age group to the following should occur approximately at the same rate in all populations with natural fertility, since it can be assumed that the natural factors affect fertility at the same rate in the various age groups. If this condition is not observed, in other words, if the slope of the fertility curve of the population with lower fertility is more rapid, it is a sign that the decline of fertility from one age to another is the consequence of a voluntary restriction of fertility, and not the influence of natural factors.

The distinction may not be as clearcut as stated above. In fact, the natural factors affecting fertility can be age-selective, and affect the younger age groups more than the older (and vice versa). Therefore, the age structure of fertility may not be the same in populations with different levels of natural fertility. However, the data reported in the following table show that the slope of the fertility curve of the three districts is by far more rapid than that of the Hutterites, and seem to suggest that natural factors are not sufficient to explain the conspicuous differences in the age structure of fertility.

Ages	*Hutterites ASMFR*	*20-24=100*	*Three districts, 1930 ASMFR*	*20-24=100*	*Three districts as percent of the Hutterites 20-24=100*
20-24	.550	100	.466	100	85
25-29	.502	91	.377	81	75
30-34	.447	81	.308	66	69
35-39	.406	74	.251	54	62
40-44	.222	40	.123	26	55
45-49	.061	11	.024	5	39

6.4. *The Hypothetical Family Size of the Districts*

Lack of space and problems of comparability have prevented us from reporting the ASMFR for the 22 districts, from 1930 to 1960. A way of summarizing this large amount of information is to compute a measure of "period" family size, or the hypothetical number of children per woman married at a given age. This measure may be obtained by summation of the ASMFR, and can be expressed (designating the marital fertility rates for the various ages as f_x and age at marriage as k) in the following way:

$$D = \sum_{k}^{50} f_x$$

In Table 33 we have reported the period family size of the districts from 1930 to 1960, for women married at age 20 and at age 25. The latter is very close to the actual age at marriage.[6] The data

[6] See note 4, Chapter 4.

Table 33. Hypothetical Number of Children per Married Woman, 1930-1960

	Mean number of children per woman married at 20				Mean number of children per woman married at 25				Percent change 1960/1930		Absolute change 1960/1930	
Districts	1930	1940	1950	1960	1930	1940	1950	1960	(4):(1)	(8):(5)	(4)−(1)	(8)−(5)
	1	2	3	4	5	6	7	8	9	10	11	12
1. Bragança	7.93	6.28	6.14	5.81	5.59	4.51	4.16	3.92	−26.7	−29.9	−2.12	−1.57
2. Vila Real	7.50	5.74	6.21	6.37	5.21	4.19	4.24	4.33	−15.1	−16.9	−1.13	− .88
3. Viana do Castelo	6.74	6.11	6.16	5.80	4.97	4.34	4.16	3.85	−14.0	−22.5	− .94	−1.12
4. Braga	7.80	6.95	7.12	7.69	5.45	5.13	4.80	5.22	− 1.4	− 4.2	− .11	− .23
5. Porto	6.20	5.30	5.68	5.70	4.01	3.42	3.65	3.60	− 8.1	−10.2	− .50	− .41
6. Guarda	6.81	6.01	5.57	5.34	4.75	4.24	3.72	3.35	−21.6	−29.5	−1.47	−1.40
7. Viseu	6.92	6.52	5.76	5.70	4.81	4.43	3.88	3.74	−17.6	−22.3	−1.22	−1.07
8. Aveiro	6.70	5.66	5.44	5.25	4.49	3.80	3.52	3.30	−21.6	−26.5	−1.45	−1.19
9. Castelo Branco	6.80	5.50	4.89	4.23	4.78	3.75	3.15	2.57	−37.8	−46.2	−2.57	−2.21
10. Coimbra	5.45	4.47	4.44	3.87	3.63	2.87	2.75	2.27	−29.0	−37.5	−1.58	−1.36
11. Leiria	6.10	5.94	4.56	4.30	4.00	3.81	2.94	2.65	−29.5	−33.7	−1.80	−1.35
12. Santarém	5.43	4.12	3.74	3.54	3.47	2.66	2.26	2.06	−34.8	−40.6	−1.89	−1.41
13. Lisbon	3.69	2.60	2.73	2.92	2.19	1.47	1.58	1.62	−20.9	−26.0	−0.77	− .57
14. Portalegre	5.68	4.21	3.40	3.19	3.54	2.72	2.05	1.80	−43.8	−49.2	−2.49	−1.74
15. Évora	5.10	4.33	3.41	3.02	3.37	2.78	2.13	1.63	−40.8	−51.6	−2.08	−1.74
16. Setúbal	4.60	3.26	2.60	2.61	2.90	2.06	1.49	1.39	−43.3	−52.1	−1.99	−1.51
17. Beja	5.51	5.27	4.16	3.75	3.74	3.55	2.73	2.21	−32.0	−40.9	−1.76	−1.53
18. Faro	4.26	3.44	2.90	2.65	2.68	2.12	1.66	1.42	−37.8	−47.0	−1.61	−1.26
19. Angra	6.13	5.29	5.25	5.67	3.83	3.73	3.52	3.68	− 7.5	− 3.9	− .46	− .15
20. Horta	5.57	4.31	4.12	3.72	3.54	2.87	2.66	2.21	−33.2	−37.6	−1.85	−1.33
21. Ponta Delgada	6.97	6.40	6.87	7.34	4.69	4.18	4.48	4.77	+ 5.3	+10.2	+ .37	+ .08
22. Funchal	8.13	6.88	7.49	7.22	5.52	4.94	5.18	4.98	−11.2	− 9.8	− .91	− .54
Portugal	5.94	4.91	4.75	4.62	3.95	3.27	3.05	2.87	−22.2	−27.3	−1.32	−1.08

validate what has been observed several times in the course of this and of the last chapter; there is a relatively weak decline, between 1930 and 1960 in the districts of the north and of the islands, a decline not exceeding 30 percent (with the exception of Horta); on the other hand a rapid fall of fertility can be observed in the south—Castelo Branco, Santarém, and the districts south of the Tagus—with a percentage change of around 40-50.

Between 1930 and 1960, according to our data, there is a decline at the national level of family size equal to 1.1 children per woman married at age 25; most of the districts of the north and of the islands have experienced a decline below the national norm; the contrary happens in the south (Figures 7a and 7b). But even more interesting is the analysis of the territorial levels of family size; in the following table the mean values for the north, the center, the south, and the islands are reported, 1930 and 1960 (women married at age 25). In 1930, the gap between north and south was already ample and evident, but in 1960 it has widened, and to the

	1930	*1960*
North	4.91	3.91
Center	3.61	2.23
South	3.20	1.69
Islands	4.40	3.91

large family size of the north (almost 4 children per woman) corresponds with the neomalthusian and regressive pattern of the south (1.7). In 1960, the center is close to the south, the islands identical to the north.

Returning to Table 33, in 1960, in five districts, including 30 percent of the population of continental Portugal, less than two children would be born to the average family at the end of the reproductive period; it can be estimated that in at least 8 districts (44 percent of the continental population) fertility was below replacement.

The peculiarity of the Portuguese fertility is self-evident; in 1960, within a small territory, a population, homogeneous as far as ethnic origin, political system, language, and religion are con-

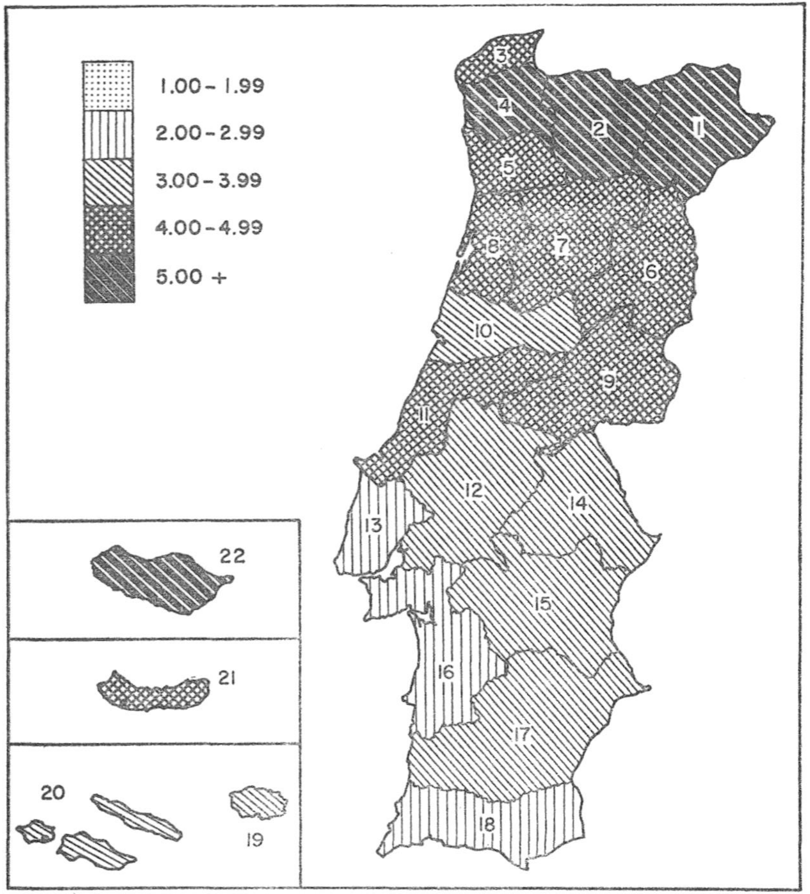

Figure 7a. Hypothetical (period) number of children per woman married at 25 years of age, 1930

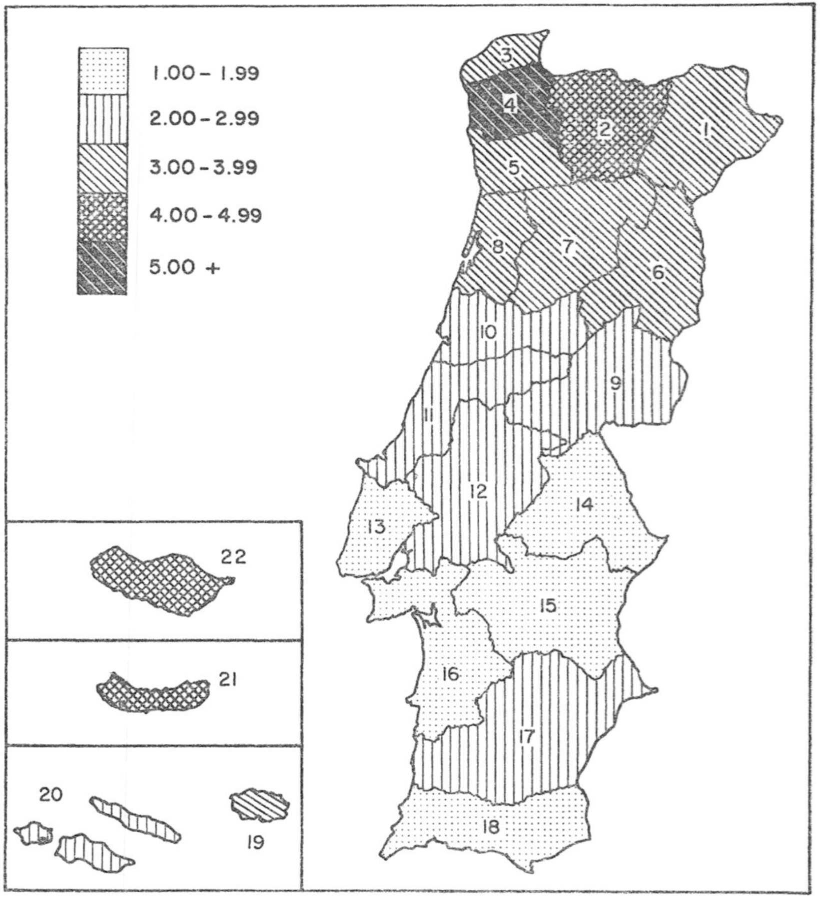

Figure 7b. Hypothetical (period) number of children per woman married at 25 years of age, 1960

cerned, exhibits both premodern patterns of fertility and neo-malthusian behavior typical of very advanced and mature societies.

6.5. *Conclusions*

The study of cohort fertility through census data, and of marital fertility by age, has added several elements of knowledge for a better understanding of Portuguese fertility. We shall attempt to summarize here the more important aspects of the statistical evidence assembled in the preceding pages.

(1) First of all, family size: The mean number of children per married woman over 45 years of age with at least 20 years of married life was 5.2 in 1940 and 3.9 in 1960. In 1940, only the selected group of women, married at 20 years of age or thereabout, and located in a few districts of the north and of the islands, had an average number of children of around 7. Even for this group, however, the completed family size is too low to be easily reconciled with a pattern of uncontrolled fertility.

(2) Cohort data drawn from the 1950 census reveal the existence of conspicuous differences of family size for the older cohorts, who had been born before 1885 and had almost completed their family size by the end of the First World War. This agrees quite well with the differences noted in I_g in 1890, 1900, and 1911.

(3) By 1960, fertility differences, expressed in terms of the hypothetical number of children per woman married at age 25, are indeed striking, extending from a minimum of 1.4 in Faro and Setúbal, to a maximum of 5.2 in Braga and 5.0 in Madeira. Similar variations cannot be found elsewhere in Europe, as far as we know, not even in Italy, Spain, and Yugoslavia, where regional contrasts, in terms of social, economic, and ethnical characteristics, appear far deeper.

(4) There is a remarkable consistency between the fertility measures derived from the census data and "period" measures based on current vital statistics.

(5) Sterility appears to be, in certain selected groups, very close to the biological level.

(6) Finally, the analysis of the census data and of the ASMFR confirm that the populations of certain areas of the north (and of the islands), still in their predecline period in recent times, had a family size far below that observed in other premodern societies. The explanation of this difference cannot be found in biological factors, since sterility in the Portuguese provinces was very low, and the breast-feeding period (Minho) was short.

Chapter 7: Factors Involved in Portugal's Fertility Decline

7.1. *Problems of Method*

Demographers know how hard it is, for several reasons, to attempt to determine the factors accounting for a decline in fertility. In the first place, we are often forced to deal with very aggregated data; the varying unit—when studying the interrelationships between fertility and other socioeconomic variables—is generally the population of a certain area, instead of the individual couple. Therefore, the independent variables which demographers are forced to correlate with fertility are the social, economic, educational characteristics of the population of each area, which have to be measured by means of percentages, rates, or ratios. We are often tempted to extend to individuals those relationships found between the "average" characteristics of each area and the correspondent level of fertility. For example, if the level of fertility of each area is positively related to the average illiteracy of each area, we are led to extend this relationship to the individuals and to assume that fertility is higher the lower the educational level of the couple. Statistical theory has pointed out that the methods for studying relationships between the characteristics of individuals have limited applicability to relationships between the characteristics of populations.

A second, important point is that many factors are likely to be involved in a fertility decline—social, economic, religious, cultural, physiological, and biological—but only a few have been recorded in the available statistics.

Finally, it is likely that the impact of each factor affecting fertility is changing according to the stage of demographic development. In other words, education e.g., may play a very important role in determining the level of fertility at the beginning of the process of fertility decline because it facilitates the diffusion of birth control knowledge through the population; but education may be irrelevant when fertility has already reached a moderate level, while other factors acquire importance. This fact may obscure the sense and the meaning of territorial, cross-sectional correlation analysis, leading to mistaken conclusions.

In spite of the difficulties just mentioned, this method is often the only one open to demographers when we study historically the interrelationships linking fertility to other variables; and in spite of its shortcomings and pitfalls, this is the method we will follow in this chapter. As a first step, however, we will study the influence of urban residence on fertility. Census data and current vital statistics offer the opportunity to measure the fertility of the urban population as such, as compared with the fertility of the population living in the rural areas. This particular aspect of our study, however, escapes the general criticism advanced earlier of the study of the relationships between the characteristics of populations.

7.2. *The Urban Population of Portugal*

The history of urban Portugal is, until recent times, the history of Lisbon and Porto, the only two large cities of the country, the poles of attraction and repulsion of the more developed areas of Portugal, between the Tagus and the Douro. It is only in Lisbon and Porto that the traditional problems of urbanism—such as overpopulation, overcrowding of slums, bad sanitary conditions, pauperism, difficulties of integration of immigrants—can be found with increasing gravity. In 1911, excluding these two cities, no other continental cities exceeded the figure of 30,000 inhabitants; there were three such in 1940 (Setúbal, Coimbra, and Vila Nova de Gaia—this last practically a suburb of Porto) and five more in 1960, of which three are suburbs of Lisbon, one of Porto, and only one an old urban center of any importance—Braga.[1]

Besides the cities mentioned above, other centers of medium sizes can by no means be considered urban, since the prevailing organization of the society and the way of life are predominantly rural, and their economy is based on agriculture.

[1] For a summary history of urbanism in Portugal, see A. Amorim Girão, "Origens e evolução do urbanismo em Portugal," *R.C.E.D.*, n. 1, 1945, pp. 39-77.

If we observe the geographical distribution of cities, we will see that the more important ones are either seaports or in close relationship with the sea by way of rivers or other easy systems of communication. This is the case of course of Lisbon and Porto, and also of Setúbal and Coimbra, the only other centers that can easily be characterized as urban, with an economic structure centered on industry in the former and on the tertiary sector in the latter. In the interior, the importance of the various cities often derives from their administrative functions as capitals of the districts, or from their roles as important regional markets.[2] There are only three centers with populations above 20,000 in districts not bordering on the sea (Évora, Covilha, and Guimãraes).

In Table 34, we show the population living in the cities that are district capitals (regardless of size) and in centers with populations over 10,000, 1911 to 1960. Of the twenty-two capital cities, only eight had more than 10,000 inhabitants in 1911, while all but four

Table 34. The Urban Population of Portugal, by Area, 1911-1960 (Population expressed in thousands living in the capital cities and in the centers with a population over 10,000)

Area	1911	1940	1950	1960
	Urban population			
North	271	438	497	628
Center	484	802	908	994
South	73	173	198	261
Islands	49	94	79	86
Portugal	882	1,507	1,682	1,969
	In percent of the total			
North	9.8	12.9	13.4	16.0
Center	25.7	31.4	31.9	33.1
South	8.3	13.7	14.5	19.0
Islands	11.9	17.4	13.4	14.5
Portugal	14.7	19.4	19.8	22.1

[2] G. Ferro, "Per uno studio delle città Portoghesi," *Annali di ricerche e studi di geografia*, Vol. XIV, 1, p. 10.

exceeded this figure in 1960; all of them have been considered "urban" because of their political role. For the other centers, the figure of 10,000 can hardly be considered a reliable borderline separating the urban from the rural areas. A rapid glance at Table 34, however, clearly shows the small size and the slow growth of the urban population, even in the unrestricted sense of "urban" adopted in our analysis.

If we except the center, where the urban proportion grew from 1/4 in 1911 to 1/3 in 1960, the incidence of the urban population is very low, ranging from 8 to 12 percent in 1911 and from 14 to 19 percent in 1960. It has to be noted that the urban proportion is higher in the south than in the north, which includes Porto; this is the consequence of the different types of population settlements, already described in 3.4, dispersed in the north, and agglomerated in rural centers in the south.

A final consideration: if we separate the districts of the interior (including Beja), from the districts bordering on the sea, the striking differences in the levels of urbanization of the two areas can be readily appreciated (see Table 35); in 1960 nearly 1/3 of the littoral population was urban, against only 1/16 of the population of the interior.

Table 35. Percent of Urban Population on the Continent

Years	*Districts bordering on the sea*	*Districts of the interior*
1911	26.8	2.9
1940	28.0	5.4
1950	28.5	5.6
1960	31.0	6.3

Summing up, 2/3 to 3/4 of the total urban population, defined in the unrestricted sense adopted here, lives in the metropolitan areas of Lisbon and Porto; only part of the remaining 1/4 to 1/3 of the total dwells in genuinely urban centers (Setúbal, Coimbra), while the larger part lives in environmental conditions that share more characteristics of rural than of urban life.

7.3. *The Fertility of the Urban and of the Rural Areas (1)*

Current vital statistics offer the opportunity of measuring the fertility level of the urban areas with a few limitations that will be discussed further on.

In Table 36 we have reported the fertility and nuptiality indices (I_f, I_g, I_h, I_m) for the cities of Lisbon and Porto, and for the rest of the corresponding districts, in 1890, 1930, and 1960. The reader will note that the marital fertility of the city of Lisbon was, in 1890, substantially lower than in the rest of the district (23 percent below), while the gap between the urban center and the remaining population is less marked for Porto (less than 7 percent).[3] By 1930, the gap had increased, and the fertility of the two

Table 36. Fertility and Nuptiality Indices in the Cities of Lisbon and Porto, and in the Rest of Their Districts

	City				Rest of District				City as a percent of rest of the district			
Year	I_f	I_g	I_h	I_m	I_f	I_g	I_h	I_m	I_f	I_g	I_h	I_m
(Lisbon)												
1890[a]	.261	.441	.140	.402	.341	.572	.055	.554	76.5	77.1	254.5	72.6
1930	.174	.266	.112	.406	.312	.466	.159	.499	55.8	57.1	70.4	81.4
1960	.203	.337	.072	.504	.140	.173	.084	.625	145.0	194.8	85.7	80.6
(Porto)												
1890	.338	.609	.144	.416	.352	.660	.069	.479	96.0	92.3	208.7	86.8
1930	.218	.371	.119	.393	.353	.645	.070	.493	61.8	57.5	58.8	79.7
1960	.290	.520	.085	.471	.329	.525	.044	.591	88.1	99.0	193.2	79.7

[a] Uncorrected values.

[3] Jorge, in "Demographia e hygiene," *op. cit.*, p. 424, gives the birth rates (1895-1897) separately for the historical and overcrowded center of the city of Porto, the peripheral area, and the suburbs. The birth rates are respectively 32.5, 26.6, and 25.5. It is uncertain, however, whether the lower birth rates of the peripheral and suburban areas are imputable to the better environmental conditions and effective control of fertility of the population or to differences in the sex-age-marital status distribution.

cities was 43 percent below the level prevailing in the rest of the districts.

From 1930 to 1960, there is a marked recovery of fertility in the two cities; in 1960, the index of marital fertility (I_g) is higher in Lisbon than in the rest of the district, while in Porto marital fertility is at the same level in the two segments of the district population. The cause of this "inversion" is probably in part the nature of the birth statistics which are classified by "place of occurrence" rather than by "place of residence." Therefore it is likely that many women who do not live in the cities of Porto and Lisbon give birth there because of the better medical organization, thus distorting the computation of fertility rates.[4]

A second way of determining rural-urban differentials has been followed by Casa Nova,[5] who has computed several measures of fertility separately for areas with a marked urban or rural character, both in the north and in the south. The urban areas are formed by those *concelhos* having, at the 1950 census, less than 20 percent of the labor force engaged in the primary sector; these include 12 *concelhos* of the Porto region in the north, and an equal number of *concelhos* around Lisbon and Setúbal in the south. The rural areas include those *concelhos* with over 80 percent of the labor force engaged in the primary sector, which form an almost contiguous area in the north (with *concelhos* of Minho, Tras-os-Montes and Beira Alta), and four groups in the south (Estremadura, Ribatejo, Alentejo, and Alentejo-Algarve). A few summary results of the study are presented in Table 37; unfortunately only measures of general fertility have been computed.[6] In spite of

[4] A similar situation occurs in regard to mortality. For recording deaths in the cities of Lisbon, Porto, and Coimbra, the Instituto Nacional de Estatística has used the double classification of place of occurrence and place of residence. In 1950, of a total of 10,243 deaths, 8,866 were deaths of residents of Lisbon. The figures for Porto are 4,833 and 4,514, and for Coimbra 1,324 and 999.

[5] A. Casa Nova, "Aspectos demográficos da população Portuguesa," *R.C.E.D.*, n. 10, pp. 7-31.

[6] The tabulation of births by place of occurrence rather than by place of residence of the mother should not greatly affect the fertility rates. Actually, the northern and southern urban areas include Porto and Lisbon, each with 11 surrounding *concelhos*, forming two large metropolitan areas. Now it is likely that most of the nonresident mothers delivering babies in Porto's and Lisbon's hospitals

Table 37. Fertility in Selected Urban and Rural Concelhos 1950-1951

	Urban		Rural		Urban as percent of rural	
	North	South	North	South	North	South
Concelhos (number)	12	12	26	22	--	--
Concelhos (pop. 000)	865	1194	447	338	--	--
Birth rate	29	16	29	21	100	76
General fertility rate	143	53	121	86	118	62
Percent of illegitimate	10	25	7	28	143	89
Gross reproduction rate	1.70	0.85	2.02	1.42	84	60

Source: Case Nova, "Aspectos Demográficos da População Portuguesa."

this limitation, the results are of relevant interest: in the north, urban and rural fertility are almost equal. It is likely, however, that the differences in marital fertility are also not large, since the higher illegitimacy of the urban population is probably compensated for significantly by the lower proportion, typical of the cities of married people (see in Table 36 the values of I_m for the city of Porto and the rest of the district).

In the south, the picture is radically different; fertility is 25 to 40 percent lower in the urban area, according to the measure employed; the gross reproduction rate is well below unity, while it barely exceeds replacement level in the rural population. Finally, a useful comparison can be made between north and south. The urban northern population has a fertility approximately double the southern urban; northern rural fertility exceeds by 40 percent the southern rural. Summing up, rural-urban differentials are irrelevant in the north, conspicuous in the south; but by far more important seems to be the gap separating the north from the south, both in "urban" and "rural" behavior. The geographical "location"

come mostly from the nearby *concelhos* already included in the metropolitan areas. On the other side, the rural areas, both in the north and in the south, are very isolated areas where the great majority of births are delivered at home.

of the population—south or north—seems to be a more important factor in determining the fertility level than the rural or urban character of the population.

7.4. *The Fertility of the Urban and of the Rural Areas (2)*

The fertility surveys of 1940, 1950, and 1960, give us some help in the analysis of rural-urban fertility differentials. In Table 38 we have reported the average number of children ever born per married woman 40-44 and 45 years and over (duration of marriage over 20 years) in each district (data already presented in Table 25) and in each district capital. If we consider the older generation (45 years and over), the fertility of the capital city is only in a few instances substantially lower than in the district.[7] The cities of Lisbon, Aveiro, Santarém, and Funchal have a fertility level 18 to 12 percent below the fertility of the corresponding districts. In the other capital cities the fertility level does not diverge substantially from the district average, exceeding it in nine instances and remaining below in eight. The mean difference between the fertility of the capital and the district is −2.8 percent, and the median is −1.17.

As for the younger generation (women from 40 to 44 years of age), the difference between the fertility of the capital city and the fertility of the whole district exceeds 10 percent in Porto, Aveiro, Lisbon, Coimbra, Ponta Delgada, and Funchal. In the other sixteen districts, the fertility of the capital exceeds the fertility of the district in five instances, and in eleven instances, remains below. The mean difference is −6.21 percent and the median −5.1 percent.

On the whole, the urban environment has a visible impact on fertility in the two large cities of the country, and particularly in Lisbon. Here, the fertility of the city was substantially lower than

[7] In Table 38, the value of 6.08 for the city of Porto appears to be too high, especially when compared with the values reported in Table 39. The different fertility of the cohorts born before 1895 cannot be explained either by the different dates of observation (Table 38, 1940 census; Table 39, 1950 census) or by the different universe (1940 currently married, and 1950 ever-married women).

Table 38. Fertility of the Districts and of the Capital Cities According to the 1940 Census

District		Average number of children ever born (duration of marriage 20 years and more) to married women					
		40-44 years			45 and over		
		district (1)	capital city (2)	percent difference 2/1 (3)	district (1)	capital city (2)	percent difference 2/1 (3)
1. Bragança		6.87	6.49	− 5.5	6.09	5.93	− 2.6
2. Vila Real		6.60	6.36	− 3.6	6.06	6.09	+ 6.5
3. Viana do Castelo		5.78	6.24	+ 8.0	5.49	5.71	+ 4.0
4. Braga		7.13	6.99	− 2.0	6.20	6.30	+ 1.6
5. Porto		5.56	3.85	−30.8	6.05	6.08	+ 0.5
6. Guarda		6.19	6.43	+ 3.9	5.75	5.81	+ 0.9
7. Viseu		5.93	5.49	− 7.4	5.55	5.25	− 5.4
8. Aveiro		5.65	4.61	−18.6	5.44	4.53	−16.8
9. Castelo Branco		5.67	5.59	− 1.4	5.60	5.47	− 2.3
10. Coimbra		4.57	3.94	−13.8	4.42	4.09	− 7.5
11. Leiria		5.29	5.71	+ 7.9	4.88	5.34	+ 9.4
12. Santarém		4.51	4.09	− 9.3	4.55	4.10	−11.8
13. Lisbon		3.71	3.15	−15.1	3.75	3.09	−17.6
14. Portalegre		4.85	4.87	+ 0.2	5.04	5.04	0.0
15. Évora		5.26	4.95	− 5.9	5.08	4.86	− 4.3
16. Setúbal		5.00	4.59	− 8.2	5.06	4.86	− 4.0
17. Beja		5.55	5.38	− 4.9	5.10	5.25	+ 2.9
18. Faro		4.21	3.85	− 8.5	4.59	4.46	− 2.8
19. Angra		5.81	6.11	+ 5.2	6.12	6.86	+12.1
20. Horta		5.37	4.99	− 7.1	5.52	5.54	+ 0.4
21. Ponta Delgada		6.97	6.07	−12.9	6.61	6.01	− 9.1
22. Funchal		7.16	6.42	−10.3	6.86	6.01	−12.4
Portugal	mean	5.63	5.28	− 6.2	5.45	5.30	− 2.8
	median	5.66	5.43	− 5.1	5.50	5.44	− 1.1

in the rest of the district by 1890, before the onset at the national level of fertility decline. In the rest of the country, fertility evolves in the capital cities and in the districts in the same way, and the decline appears to be only slightly accelerated in the capital cities.

The rapid decline of fertility from one generation to the following one can easily be appreciated in Table 39, where the average

Table 39. Average Number of Children per Ever-married Woman, 1950 Census

	Cohort of Birth				1875 = 100			
	–1875	1875-1885	1885-1895	1895-1905	–1875	1875-1885	1885-1895	1895-1905
City of Porto	4.07	3.76	3.27	2.85	100	92.4	80.3	70.0
Rest of district	5.29	5.14	5.01	4.61	100	97.2	94.7	87.1
City/rest of dist.	76.9	73.2	65.3	61.8	--	--	--	--
City of Lisbon	3.57	3.01	2.55	2.20	100	84.3	71.4	61.6
Rest of district	4.35	4.33	4.08	3.51	100	99.5	93.8	80.7
City/rest of dist.	82.1	69.5	62.5	62.7	--	--	--	--

number of children ever born per ever-married woman is reported for the cities of Lisbon and Porto (1950 census; see also 6.2, Table 28). In Porto, the family size declines from 4.07 for the cohort born before 1875, to 2.85 for the cohort born at the turn of the century (1895-1905); in Lisbon the decline between the two cohorts is from 3.6 to 2.2. It is interesting to note that the older cohorts had, in both cities, a relatively modest family size, evident sign of the diffusion of voluntary restriction of procreation well before the end of the century. Secondarily, the fertility of the population living in the cities declines more rapidly than the fertility of the women living in the rest of the districts, although the starting point is lower in the former than in the latter.

A final documentation on rural-urban differentials is offered by Table 40, where the average number of children ever born per married woman (1960 fertility survey, see 6.2, Table 29) is re-

Table 40. Average Number of Children Ever Born per Married Woman, Urban and Rural Population, 1960 Census

Age at marriage \ Age at census	-20	20-24	25-29	30-34	35-39	40-44	45-49	50+	Total
				Urban population					
-20	.65	1.37	2.04	2.43	2.71	2.95	3.13	3.59	2.51
20-24	--	.71	1.39	1.96	2.28	2.49	2.57	2.91	2.11
25-29	--	--	.77	1.42	1.81	2.02	2.17	2.38	1.82
30-34	--	--	--	.94	1.43	1.67	1.82	1.98	1.66
35-39	--	--	--	--	1.06	1.41	1.54	1.70	1.53
40-44	--	--	--	--	--	1.14	1.31	1.49	1.40
45-49	--	--	--	--	--	--	1.14	1.45	1.39
50+	--	--	--	--	--	--	--	1.49	1.49
Total	.65	.92	1.34	1.78	2.07	2.23	2.29	2.51	2.01
				Rural population					
-20	.58	1.58	2.55	3.37	4.06	4.65	5.01	5.30	3.57
20-24	--	.84	1.77	2.74	3.48	4.09	4.37	4.69	3.32
25-29	--	--	.95	1.98	2.78	3.42	3.74	4.10	3.11
30-34	--	--	--	1.24	2.04	2.75	3.03	3.40	2.83
35-39	--	--	--	--	1.56	2.11	2.32	2.68	2.42
40-44	--	--	--	--	--	1.79	1.92	2.11	2.04
45-49	--	--	--	--	--	--	2.05	1.99	2.00
50+	--	--	--	--	--	--	--	2.39	2.39
Total	.58	1.10	1.77	2.56	3.22	3.76	4.00	4.20	3.22
				Rural as percent of urban					
-20	89.2	115.3	125.0	138.7	149.8	157.6	160.1	147.6	142.2
20-24	--	118.3	127.3	139.8	152.6	164.3	170.0	161.2	157.3
25-29	--	--	123.4	139.4	153.6	169.3	172.4	172.3	170.9
30-34	--	--	--	131.9	142.7	164.7	166.5	171.7	170.5
35-39	--	--	--	--	147.2	149.7	150.6	157.6	158.2
40-44	--	--	--	--	--	157.0	146.6	141.6	145.7
45-49	--	--	--	--	--	--	179.8	137.2	143.9
50+	--	--	--	--	--	--	--	160.4	160.4
Total	89.2	119.6	132.1	143.8	155.6	168.6	174.7	167.3	160.2

ported (by age at marriage and age at census) by residence. The average family size of rural wives 40 to 49 years old is 70 percent larger than the family size of the urban wives of the same age group (approximately 3.5 and 2.3 children per married woman); the differences are less marked for the younger age groups (+56 percent for women aged 35-39; +32 percent for those aged 25-29 etc.).

7.5. *Territorial Variance of Fertility*

We have already pointed out that regional variability of fertility has strongly increased from the end of the nineteenth century to 1960, a consequence of the differential development of fertility, declining rapidly in the south, slowly in the north. We have also noted, at the beginning of this paper, that Portugal can be subdivided into geographical regions, each one having marked characteristics of its own; we have retained here the usual partition in north, center, south and islands.

The analysis of variance enables us to achieve the separation of the total variation of district fertility into two parts: the variation arising from the varying of the four regions around their "grand mean" and the variation arising from the varying of the districts around their regional means. The ratio of the mean square variance "between" regions to the mean square variance "within regions," or F, adequately tested, indicates whether the variation of the regional levels around the grand mean is significantly larger than the variation of the district fertility around their regional mean—or, in short, whether regional differentials in fertility are "significant" or not.

The results of the F test on I_g are given below:

1890	$P\,(F_{3,17} = 2.467) > .05$
1900	$P\,(F_{3,17} = 3.862) < .05$
1911	$P\,(F_{3,17} = 4.620) < .05$
1920	$P\,(F_{3,17} = 4.691) < .05$
1930	$P\,(F_{3,18} = 7.928) < .01$
1940	$P\,(F_{3,18} = 6.987) < .01$
1950	$P\,(F_{3,18} = 15.457) < .01$
1960	$P\,(F_{3,18} = 20.597) < .01$

Regional differentials are not significant in 1890; they are significant at the .05 level from 1900 to 1920, and at the .01 level after 1930. The value of F rapidly increases from the end of the last century, indicating the growing impact of regional patterns of fertility.

The analysis of variance may be of some help to us in solving another problem. Up to now, the analysis of fertility has been done mainly at the district level, under the assumption that the population of each district is homogeneous as far as fertility behavior is concerned. Now, it is true that the average dimensions of the districts are rather small, both in terms of population (slightly over 200,000 in 1864; twice that in 1960) and territorial extension (5,000 km^2), and are therefore adapted to a detailed demographic study; still, it has to be proved that fertility levels do not vary to a large extent within each district. Therefore, the analysis of variance has been extended to the 271 *concelhos* and the eighteen districts of the continent, and to the twenty-nine *concelhos* and four districts of the islands. The F test has been computed for the average 1930-1940 birth rate. The 1930-1940 decade has been selected because of the very rapid fall of fertility (the birth rate declines, for the whole country, from 30.2 in 1928-1932 to 25.0 in 1938-1942) and the dramatic differentiation in the attitude towards procreation of the regional populations. The results of the F test can be summarized as follows:

$$\text{1930-1940, Continent} = P\ (F_{271,17} = 13.150) < .01$$
$$\text{1930-1940, Islands} = P\ (F_{29,3} = 30.222) < .01$$

The large values of F (significant at the 0.1 level, both on the continent and on the islands) indicate that a large portion of variance is between districts, and only a small proportion within. The relative homogeneity of districts should save us from doubting the meaning of analysis of fertility at the district level rather that at the more detailed level of *concelhos.*

Analysis of variance tells us that regional differentials are significant in the statistical sense, but we are also interested in following the process of geographic differentiation of marital fertility. We had already observed that fertility tends to decrease passing from east to west and from north to south, following the lines of the historical development of the country. We have computed Spearman's rank correlation coefficient (r_r) between the order of the districts according to their geographical location and according to their fertility level (I_g). The geographical order is the one given in the tables to the Portuguese districts, from east to west and from north to south; the islands have been excluded from the computation.

The rank correlation coefficients, computed from 1890 to 1960, indicate a positive and increasing association between geographical location and the level of marital fertility. By 1960, the geographical and fertility rank orders nearly coincide, and r_r is over .900.

Rank Correlation Coefficient Between I_g and Geographical Location

1890	+.630	1930	+.853
1900	+.471	1940	+.873
1911	+.569	1950	+.892
1920	+.843	1960	+.901

If we rank the districts according to the percent decrease of I_g between 1890 and 1960, r_r is even higher, equal to .934.

Summing up the findings of this section, we may say that regional differentials, not significant in 1890, become more and more relevant as time goes by (and fertility falls), and that the diffusion of fertility control follows a precise geographical orientation, proceeding from the coast toward the interior, and from south to north.

7.6. *Social and Economic Correlates of Fertility*

It is clear by now that the Portuguese fertility decline follows a rather precise territorial pattern. This trend, however, may occur because other factors influencing the level of fertility make their impact felt in a spreading movement proceeding westward or southward; or because the diffusion of neomalthusianism, initiated in the south, has spread by diffusion of new attitudes and ideas to other regions in geographical order. More likely, the two interpretations coexist: neomalthusianism spreads to other areas because of geographical contiguity, but is fostered (or checked) in its diffusion by the social and economic conditions prevailing in each area.

We will examine, now, the interrelationships between fertility and a few socioeconomic variables through correlation analysis of the 1911, 1930, and 1960 data. The variables considered are infant mortality; an index of illiteracy (percent of males 25-29 who could not write or read); an index of primary activity (percent of the labor force engaged in agriculture); and, a measure of emigration (emigrants per 1,000 population). For 1960 we have added two further variables: an index of the medical organization serving the population (percent of the newborn without medical assistance) and an index of religiosity (percent of the population which was declared to be Catholic). Figures 8a to 8f show the value of socioeconomic indices for each district in 1960.

The results of the correlation analysis are reported in Table 41 (the significance of the correlation coefficients has been tested with Student's T).

Table 41. Zero Order Correlation Coefficients Between I_g and:

Year	Infant mortality	Illiteracy	Percent employed in agriculture	Emigration	Percent of births with no medical assistance	Percent Catholic
1911	+.319	+.239	+.498[b]	+.294	--	--
1930	-.090	+.204	+.566[a]	+.575[a]	--	--
1960	+.699[a]	-.163	+.123	+.656[a]	+.856[a]	+.695[a]

a = significant at the .01 level

b = significant at the .05 level

The correlation coefficients have, most of the time, the expected sign (the various indices are all expected to be positively correlated with fertility), with the exception of infant mortality in 1930 and of illiteracy in 1960.

In 1911 only the correlation coefficient between I_g and the index of primary activity is significant; in 1930 I_g is significantly correlated also with the index of emigration, and in 1960 with the

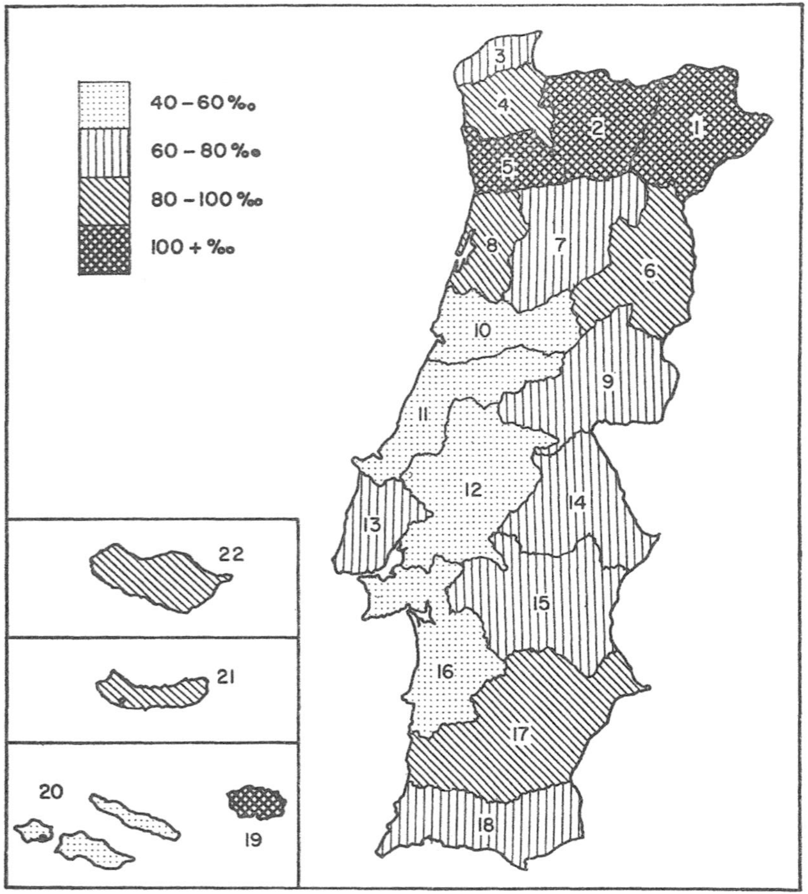

Figure 8a. Infant mortality, 1960-1962

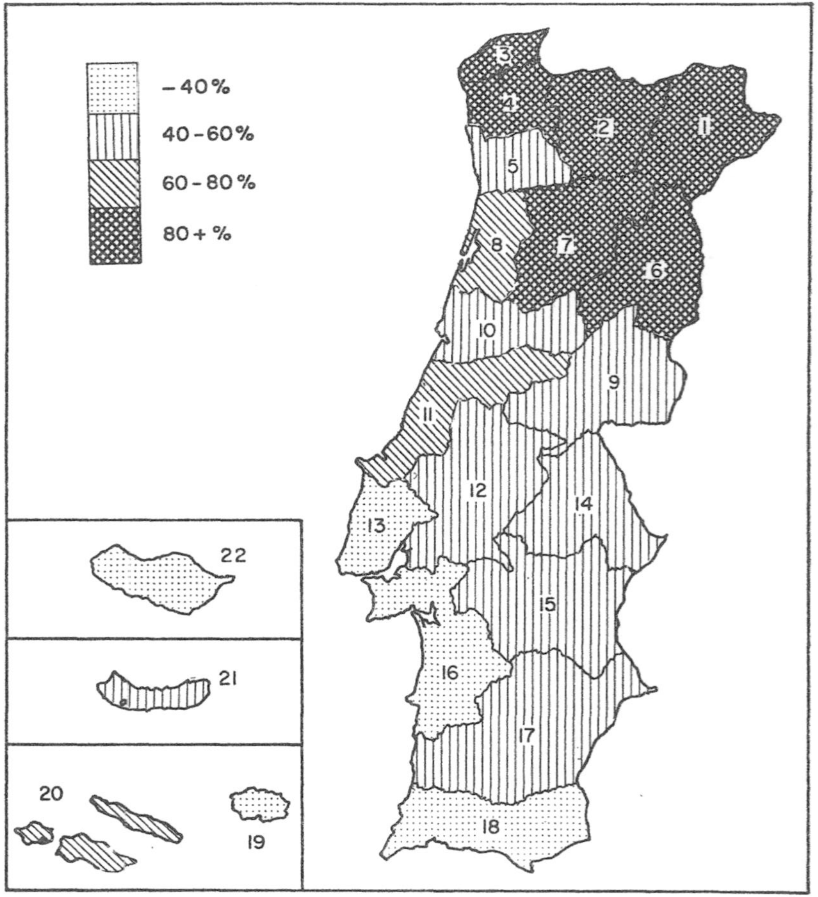

Figure 8b. Percentage of babies born without assistance, 1960

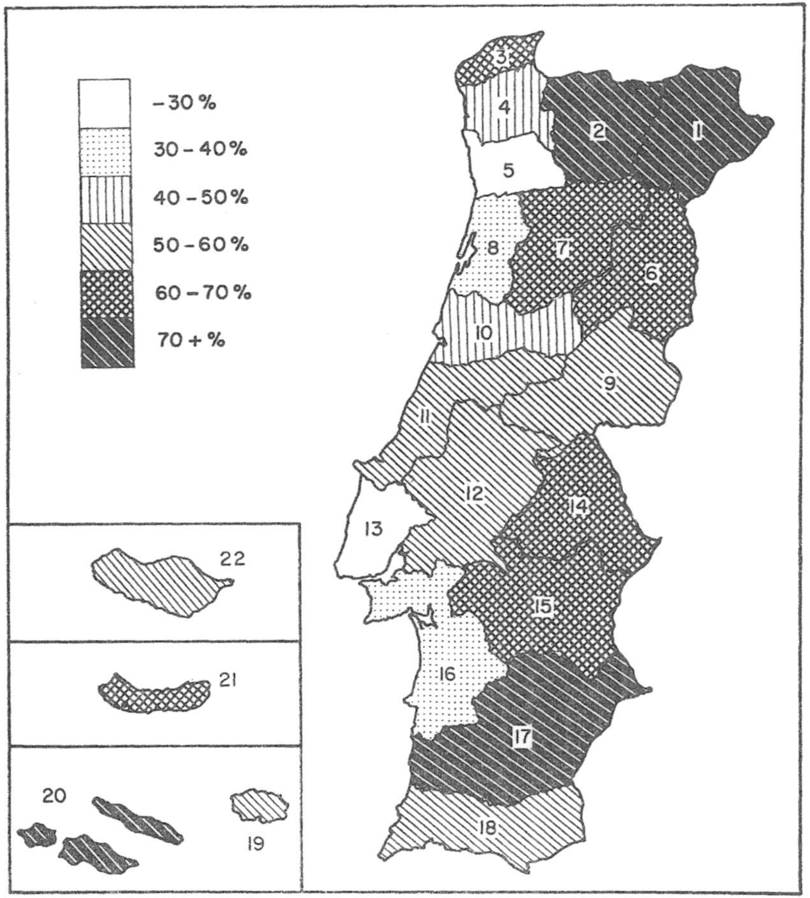

Figure 8c. Percentage of the labor force engaged in agriculture, 1960

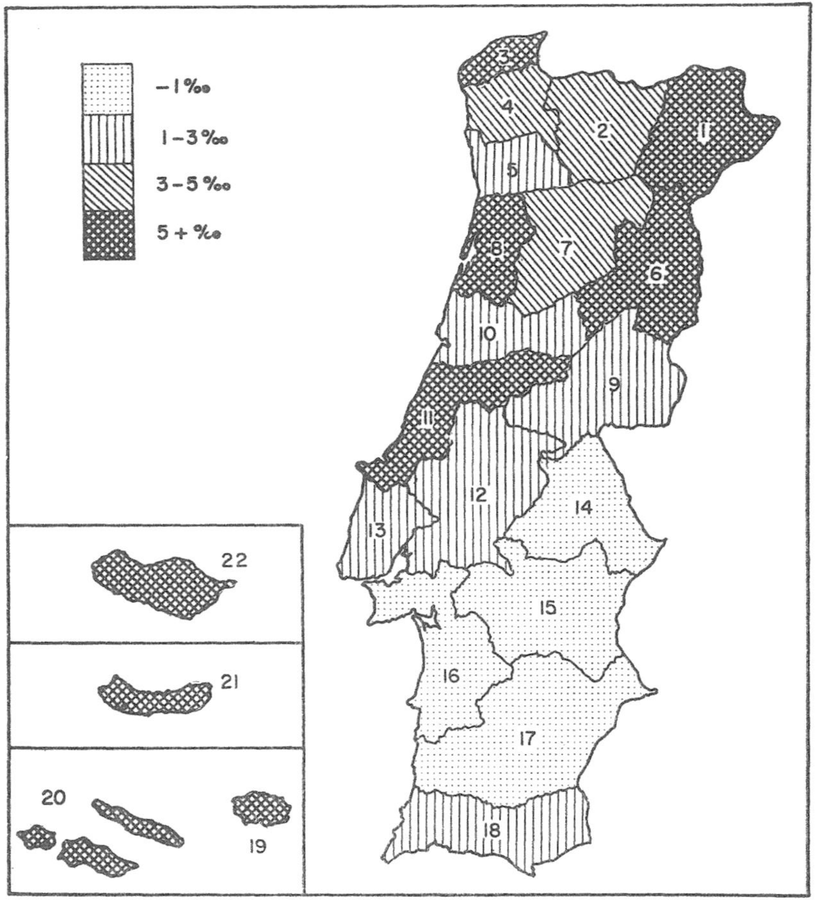

Figure 8d. Emigrants per thousand population, 1960-1962

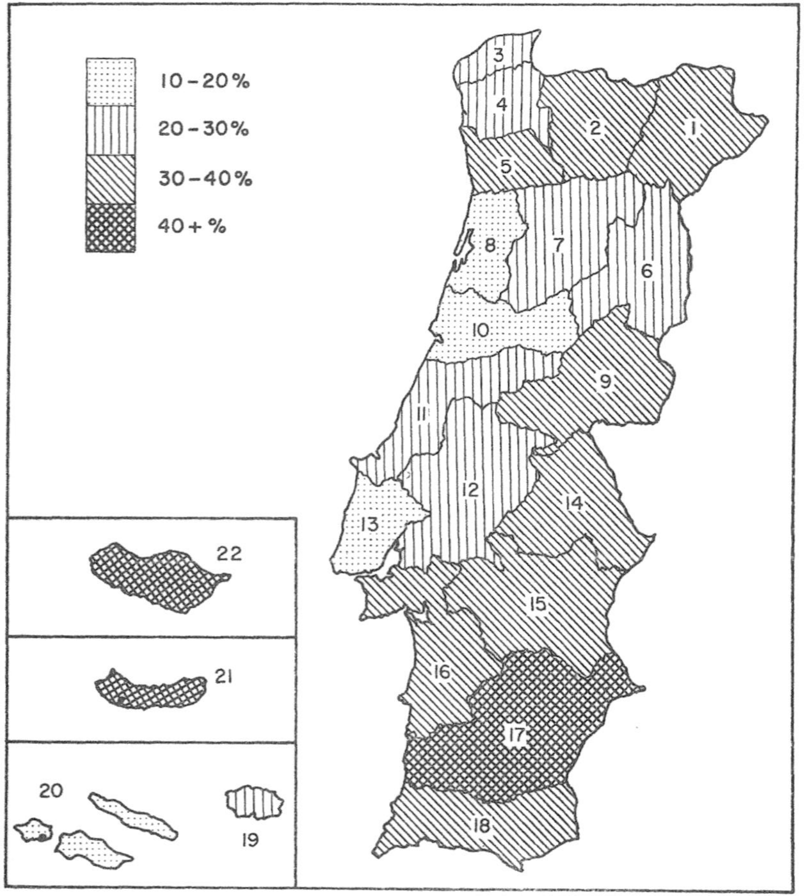

Figure 8e. Percentage illiterate among males aged 25-29, 1960

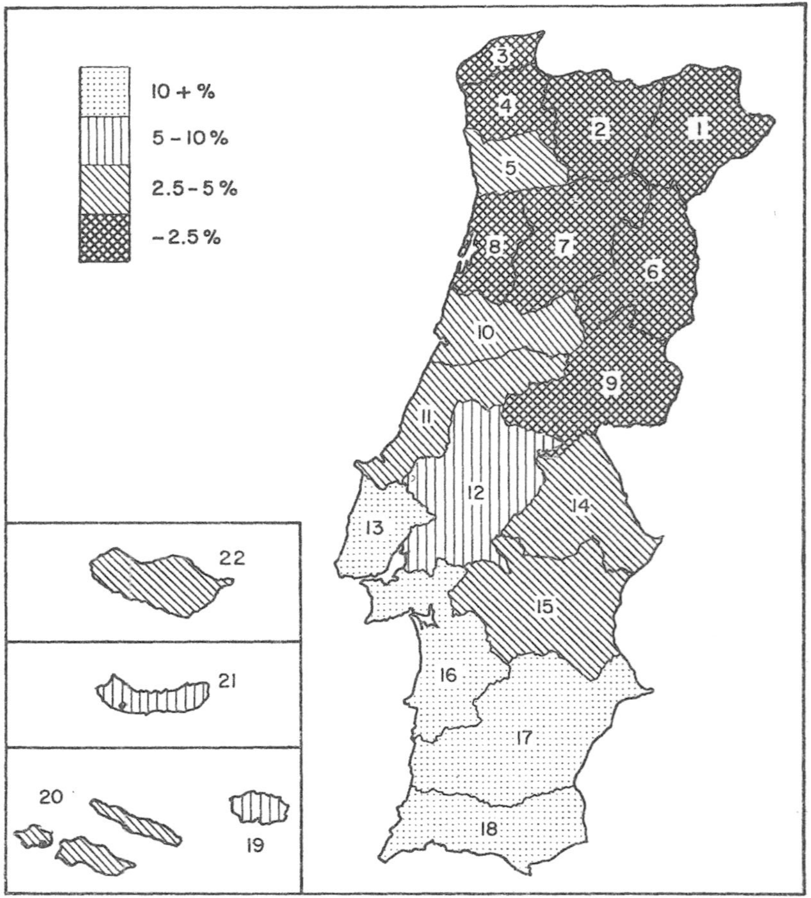

Figure 8f. Percentage of marriages celebrated without the Catholic rite, 1960

indices of infant mortality, emigration, medical facilities, and religiosity. It is interesting to note that marital fertility is never significantly associated with illiteracy, which, nevertheless, is one of the variables most frequently cited in explaining fertility differentials.

It has been observed that regional differences of marital fertility are increasingly important beginning from the first of this century. On the other hand, we have found sometimes significant correlation coefficients between fertility and some socioeconomic variables. We would like to know whether regional differences are still significant once the effects of each of the socioeconomic variables have been removed. We may get the answer we are looking for through covariance analysis, by computation of the *F* test. Practically, the *F* test tells us if the regional means of marital fertility (I_g) still differ significantly one from the other, once the effects of mortality, illiteracy, and any other variable have been removed from the regional means.

In Table 42 we have reported the values of the *F* test, together with a measure of the "degree of association" between marital fertility and regional location. The degree of association is measured by:

$$\sqrt{1 - \frac{\text{mean square variance within regions}}{\text{mean square variance, total}}}$$

With the computation of *F* and of the degree of association, we have removed from I_g, on a one-by-one basis, the effects of the four independent variables considered in this study. We have limited the analysis to 1930 and 1960, periods in which regional patterns of fertility have become more and more evident. Finally, at the foot of the table, we have reported the value of the *F* test done through the simple analysis of variance of I_g (without allowance for the effects of either one of the four variables). These last values do not coincide with those reported in 7.5, because the fourth region, including Madeira and Azores, has been here excluded from the correlation analysis.

The *F* values reported in Table 42 are always highly significant,

Table 42. Analysis of Covariance of I_g for 18 Districts and 3 Regions

Year	$F_{2,15}$	Degree of Association
a) after allowance for effect of infant mortality		
1930	12.70[a]	.762
1960	15.34[a]	.792
b) after allowance for effect of illiteracy		
1930	31.71[a]	.909
1960	41.48[a]	.912
c) after allowance for effect of percent of labor force engaged in agriculture		
1930	7.14[a]	.648
1960	34.96[a]	.894
d) after allowance for effect of emigration		
1930	5.46[b]	.587
1960	16.64[a]	.805
Analysis of variance of I_g		
1930	12.77[a]	
1960	34.51[a]	

a = significant at the .01 level

b = significant at the .05 level

both in 1930 and 1960. This means, in other words, that the removal of the effects of each "independent" variable does not account for regional differences in fertility. We might have expected this result, because the allowance for the effects of the socioeconomic variables has been done on a one-by-one rather than multiple basis, while the interrelationships between fertility and the various socioeconomic factors are complex and interdependent.

If we compare the *F* values obtained through covariance analysis with the *F* values obtained through various analysis and reported in the low section of Table 42, we see that in 1930, regional differences are "reduced" after allowance for the effects of emigration and percent engaged in agriculture; they are, on the other hand, "increased" after allowance for the effects of illiteracy, and remain unaltered after accounting for infant mortality. In 1960, regional differentials are increased after allowance for illiteracy and reduced after allowance for emigration and infant mortality.

In short, illiteracy tended to obscure, rather than to accentuate, as one might have expected, the regional differences both in 1930 and in 1960. This is, perhaps, the most striking result of the covariance analysis.

7.7. *Factors of Fertility Differentials: Partial and Multiple Correlation Analysis*

We want now to answer a different set of questions. The first one is: How close is the correlation between fertility and each one of the socioeconomic variables, once the effects of the remaining variables are accounted for? With the second question, we may ask how close is the correlation between fertility and the socioeconomic variables simultaneously taken into account? The computation of the partial and multiple correlation coefficients will enable us to answer these questions and to add an important piece of information to our analysis. We have selected three "independent" variables: the index of mortality, the index of illiteracy, and the index of primary activity, computing the partial and multiple correlation coefficients, which we have reported in Table 43. In the same table, in order to facilitate the comparison, we have reported the values of the zero-order correlation coefficients already indicated in 7.6.

The results of the analysis call for a few comments. In the first place, in 1911, 1930, and 1960 the partial correlations between I_g and the index of mortality and between I_g and the index of primary activity are higher than the correspondent zero-order coefficients. The partial coefficients, moreover, have always the expected (positive) sign, and are statistically significant. In other words, the influence of the other factors tends to obscure the existing relationship between these variables and marital fertility.

Comments of the opposite nature have to be made concerning the relationships between fertility and illiteracy. In 1911, the zero-

Table 43. Zero Order, Partial, and Multiple Correlation Coefficients Between Marital Fertility (I_g) and Three Socioeconomic Variables

Year	Type of correlation	Index of mortality	Index of illiteracy	Index of primary activity
	Zero-order	+.319	+.239	+.498
1911	Partial	+.659	+.151	+.684
	Multiple		.759	
	Zero-order	−.090	+.204	+.566
1930	Partial	+.331	−.257	+.626
	Multiple		.647	
	Zero-order	+.699	−.163	+.123
1960	Partial	+.849	−.704	+.567
	Multiple		.864	

order correlation was positive, as expected, but the partial correlation reveals an inverse relationship; in 1930 the positive partial correlation coefficient is lower than the zero-order coefficient; in 1960 the partial coefficient strengthens the inverse relationship already revealed by the zero-order correlation between the two variables. Both in 1930 and in 1960, therefore, allowance for the effects of the other variables results in the strengthening of an association contrary to any reasonable hypothesis: the higher is illiteracy, the lower is fertility and the stronger its control. The reader may be interested in the fact that in both Italy and Spain illiteracy is closely and directly associated with fertility, and indeed is the social variable most highly correlated with fertility differentials.

For 1960, we have computed partial and multiple correlation coefficients between I_g and another set of variables: emigration, the proportion of babies delivered without medical assistance, and the proportion of the population which declared itself Catholic at the 1960 census. Below are the results of the computations compared, as in Table 43, with the zero-order coefficients:

Type of correlation	*Emigration*	*Percent of babies born without medical assistance*	*Percent Catholic*
Zero-order	+.656	+.856	+.695
Partial	−.145	+.686	+.278
Multiple		.868	

Partial correlation coefficients are lower than the corresponding zero-order ones, but for the second and third variable maintain the positive sign.

Finally, the multiple correlation coefficient was lowest in 1930, explaining only 42 percent of the variance, and highest in 1960, when 75 percent of the variance is explained by either one of the two sets of three variables which have been associated with marital fertility. On the whole, fertility differentials can be explained to a large extent by the socioeconomic variables simultaneously considered, although illiteracy plays an unexpected role. A final elaboration has been attempted. We have seen earlier that after allowing (on a one-by-one basis) for the influence of the various variables, the differences between regions, far from being eliminated, are, in certain instances, increased. We may now try another form of analysis by computing, for each district, the deviation of every variable from the regional mean, then calculating the correlation between fertility and the independent variables (expressed in terms of deviations from the regional means). In this way, we may see the level of association between variables once the effects of the region in which a district is located have been removed. The results of the correlation analysis for 1930 and 1960 are reported in the following table and compared with the results contained in Table 43. Once the "regional impact" is removed, the relationships between variables are much altered and generally weaker; partial coefficients, for instance, are by far lower and mostly opposite in sign, when computed on deviations instead of on absolute values. Of particular interest is the fact that when the influence of "region" is removed, the strongest partial correlation of marital fertility is with illiteracy, and the relation is positive, as expected.

Variables	Correlation between absolute values: Zero order	Correlation between absolute values: Partial	Correlation between deviations from regional means: Zero order	Correlation between deviations from regional means: Partial
		1930		
Index of mortality	−.090	.331	−.371	−.050
" " illiteracy	.204	−.257	.702	.449
" " primary activity	.566	.626	.712	.392
		1960		
Index of mortality	.699	.849	.158	−.176
" " illiteracy	−.163	−.704	.405	.397
" " primary activity	.123	.567	.160	−.136

Although it appears evident that traditionally employed social correlates of fertility, such as mortality, illiteracy, rurality, are not the main causes of fertility differentials between regions, the interpretation of the results is not easy. Regional differences could be explained, perhaps, by other variables whose measurement is difficult (religiosity, for instance) or impossible, which concur to form the cultural and environmental conditions of every regional population. On the other hand, other factors of a mainly biological nature could also be taken into account in explaining regional differences in fertility. We have discussed the various aspects of sterility on the basis of census data. Some information on duration of breastfeeding is also available. The existing evidence on breastfeeding, however, is of a nonstatistical nature, and its possible role in determining the level of fertility will be discussed in the following pages. The whole complex problem of the determinants of fertility will be reexamined and reassessed also in the light of considerations of a nonquantitative nature, which would have been out of place in this chapter where the whole subject has been approached in a rather technical way.

Conclusion

The statistical and qualitative evidence presented and analyzed in this study calls for a final discussion and reappraisal of the principal findings.

One of the more interesting aspects of Portuguese demography is the relatively low level of fertility before the start of the modern decline, together with the existence, during the same period, of substantial differences between north and south. The marital fertility of Portuguese women never exceeded 70 percent of the fertility of the Hutterites, a performance well in line with the patterns existing in Spain and in Italy before the end of the nineteenth-century. The fertility of the north, however, was, during the same period, substantially higher than that of the south; the mean value of I_g in 1890 was sixteen percent above the southern level, while the mean number of children per currently married woman born before 1895 was 17 percent higher. The mean number of children per ever-married woman born before the same date was 9 to 12 percent higher.

The reasons for the relatively low level of premodern Portuguese fertility are, of course, not clear. Sterility was generally very low; childless women who had almost completed their fecund period (1940) and had married around twenty years of age, accounted for only 2 to 5 percent of the total (with the exceptions only of Lisbon and Beja), a level of sterility very close to the biological minimum. On the other hand, breastfeeding was probably universal, and was generally prolonged well into the second year of life of the child. Portuguese ethnologist Vasconcellos collected information about the breastfeeding habits of regional populations (see Table 44). According to Vasconcellos, there are frequent cases of children of 2 to 3 years who are still breastfed by mothers. The duration and the diffusion of breastfeeding habits may be one of the factors of the relatively long intervals between births, although we are confident that the modest level of premodern fertility was also the consequence of diffusion to a certain extent of voluntary control on procreation. Still, the reasons for the differ-

Table 44. Duration(in Months) of Breastfeeding by Area

Area	Normal duration	Maximum duration
Lisbon (Estremadura)	8 - 12	20 and over
Estremoz (Alto Alentejo)	12 - 16	24
Amarante (Minho)	12 - 15	24 - 50
Gafete (Alto Alentejo)	14 and over	--
Guarda (Beira)	12 - 14	--
Tras-os-Montes	24 - 30	--
Minho	18	--

Source: Leite de Vasconcellos, Etnografia Portuguesa, Vol. 4, Lisbon, 1958, pp. 458-460.

ences between north and south are not clear, but can be imputed neither to the impact of sterility nor to divergent breastfeeding habits. It is interesting to note here that as early as the eighteenth-century the notion of higher fertility among the women of the Minho was widespread in contemporary writers; Rebelo da Costa observed that "women of the Minho are the most fertile of the Kingdom. Even if we do not go back to ancient times, nowadays many women live who have borne 25 children, and some of them even 30."[1] Bautista da Castro said, "its inhabitants [of the Minho] have a very high reproductivity and long life."[2]

A further important finding of our research is the relevance of between-region fertility differences which persist and are even accentuated when other factors are accounted for. Moreover, the association between fertility and other social correlates, although in many instances close and significant, is not always as expected; illiteracy, for instance, is inversely correlated with fertility. When we allow for the effect of regional similarity, most correlations are reduced, and the usual positive relationship with illiteracy is revealed as prevalent.

[1] A. Rebelo da Costa, *Descripção topográfica e historica da cidade do Porto*, Porto, 1788, p. xvii.

[2] Quoted by J. Leite de Vasconcellos, *Etnografia Portuguesa,* Vol. IV, Lisbon, 1958, p. 456.

The existence of remarkable regional differences calls for a few interesting reflections. In the first place, it has to be remembered that regional differences in fertility can be found also in the other Mediterranean countries: in Italy, where the marital fertility of the south is 60-70 percent higher than in the north; in Yugoslavia, where the south (Macedonia, Kosovo) has a fertility far higher than the north (Croatia, Serbia); in Spain, where the neomalthusian northeast can be opposed to the still prolific south. In these countries, however, the low fertility areas are, by far, the more developed from the social and economic point of view, as is revealed by any one of the indices commonly used for the purpose of measuring the standard of living of a population. Italy is the most evident case, since the contrast between the north and the south is clear-cut and dates back to old times; but in Yugoslavia and in Spain the differences in the standard of living between the neomalthusian and the prolific populations are also evident.

This is not the case in Portugal. There is no evident difference between the standard of living of the north and of the south (from which is excluded, let us recall, the district of Lisbon); on the contrary, by many of the more commonly used standards, the south appears more backward than the north. For a better appraisal of the north-south differentials, we have reported in Table 45, the regional means of fertility and of other indices.

As Table 45 clearly shows, the south has more illiteracy, more labor force engaged in agriculture, is less industrialized, and has a lower participation of women in economic activities. By these standards, the south appears more backward than the north. On the other hand, the north is less urbanized, has a much higher infant mortality rate, a higher death rate for infectious diseases (and therefore a worse sanitary system), and a much higher external migration. The least we can say is that neither one of the two populations can claim to be privileged with an incontestable higher standard of living.

Still, the two populations are deeply differentiated. Variable 11 indicates that in the north very small farm holdings prevail and are partly responsible for the high emigration rate; in the south—

Table 45. Regional Means of Fertility and Other Indices for the North and the South

	Variables	North	South	South as percent of the north
	Marital Fertility (I_g)	.539	.255	47
1.	Illiteracy (males, 25-29)	27.9	37.8	136
2.	Population density (Km^2)	166.0	45.0	27
3.	Percent urban population	16.0	19.0	84
4.	Percent of labor force engaged in agriculture	56.7	58.0	102
5.	Percent of labor force engaged in manufacturing	17.7	15.2	86
6.	Percent of females in the labor force	17.9	14.1	79
7.	Infant mortality	91.5	69.6	76
8.	Death rate (100,000) from infectious diseases	100.2	68.5	68
9.	Percent of babies born without assistance	77.4	44.0	52
10.	Emigration rate (per thousand)	4.9	.8	16
11.	Average size (ha) of farm holding	2.1	26.2	1248
12.	Percent of marriages performed without Catholic rite	1.5	14.4	960

as in Andalusia and in Spanish Estremadura—the land is concentrated in a few latifundia (with the exception of the Algarve), and farm laborers constitute a large percentage of the agricultural labor force. Still the large estate system, although deeply differentiating the south from the north, can hardly be thought as a factor of low fertility, being generally associated with rather primitive living conditions and—as in Italy and Spain—with a large family system.

There is little doubt that it is at least awkward to decide which region—the north or the south—is more advanced from a social and economic point of view. The traditionally invoked association between fertility and mortality, industrialization, urbanization, or literacy fails to give unequivocal results in the Portuguese case. The contrast between north and south cannot be satisfactorily explained by any one of the above mentioned variables. But the demographer and the sociologist willing to give an interpretation of complex phenomena such as fertility have to be free from the fear that "quod non est in numero non est in mundo." There are certainly other factors, which cannot be measured statistically but nevertheless are not less important, at the base of the different behavior of the north and of the south. Among these factors, religiosity is certainly a powerful one. Variable 12 clearly shows that the south is more secularized and less observant of rites than the north; in the south the relatively large proportion of marriages not performed according to the Catholic rite and the high fraction of the population declaring themselves non-Catholic at the 1960 census (but not belonging to other confessions) reveals the diffusion of an attitude radically different from that prevailing in the north. The north (particularly the Minho region) is well known, on the other hand, for its religiosity and deep attachment to the Church's precepts. The reader has already been repeatedly informed as to the different regional attitudes toward religion (see 1.5 and 4.3). It could be thought that the south, with more secular attitudes, has been receptive to the neomalthusian principles, while the north's religiosity and deep attachment to traditions may have erected efficient barriers to the diffusion of voluntary control of fertility. Vasconcellos has given several elements for judging religious observance in the various regions. Says Vasconcellos, "in spite of the efforts of the clergy in order to maintain the purity of the faith, I would say that—according to the information I have collected, in many instances by the clergy itself, and to what can be observed at any step—the Alentejo is the region which least practices religion."[3] In the opinion of Vasconcellos, the Alentejano is not only indifferent but also irreverent towards religion and its precepts—a mentality often caused by the isolation of the rural populations, the rarity of clergymen, and the semi-nomadic structure of internal

[3] Vasconcellos, *op. cit.*, Vol. III, Lisbon, 1942, p. 524.

seasonal migrations.[4] A rapid decline of religiosity is observed by the same author, particularly in the urban areas, in Estremadura and Algarve.[5]

All that is in contrast with the deep attachment to Catholicism of the populations of the north, and particularly of the Minho; in the words of Sampaio "religiosity is the base of the moral life of the Minhotos. They walk for miles in order to listen to the sermon of a famous preacher."[6] The separation of Church and state after 1911 further differentiated the south from the north. An investigation of the government into popular reactions to the separation showed the irritation and opposition of the northerners and the passive acceptance of the southerners. But the popular reactions could be more dramatically judged by the frequency of riots against the new order in the north, and the many cases of anticlerical intolerance in the south.[7]

Religiosity is only a component, although a powerful one, of the cultural world of a population. In the Minho, religiosity goes along with a widespread attachment to traditions, with a strong family life, with an obedient attitude towards any kind of authority, with a patient and enduring character, and with an innate suspicion of innovation.

Many Portuguese writers, on the other hand, observe that the irreligiosity of the south goes along with the passivity and indolence of its people, with its moral indifference, with the weakness of family ties.[8]

All that may not be sufficient to explain the different regional attitudes towards procreation, and may not satisfy all those who look for exactly measurable cause-and-effect relationships between demographic and social, economic and cultural variables. But it is

[4] *Ibid.*, pp. 524-526.

[5] *Ibid.*, pp. 406-407, 618.

[6] A. Sampaio, *Estudos históricos e económicos,* Vol. I, Porto, 1923, pp. 530-534 (quoted by Vasconcellos, *op. cit.*, Vol. IV, p. 565).

[7] Vasconcellos, *op. cit.*, Vol. IV, see the paragraph "Religiosidade dos Portugueses," pp. 508-522.

[8] See also the conclusion drawn by Ribeiro at the end of Vol. IV of Vasconcellos' *Etnografia Portuguesa*, published posthumously in 1958, pp. 630ff.

also true that almost everywhere attachment to traditions and loyalty to religion—to Catholic religion—go along with a slow acceptance of fertility control, in Ireland as in the Netherlands, in Italy as in Switzerland. Should we expect Portugal to be an exception?

Appendix

Underregistration and Adjustment of Births

In sections 3.2. and 3.3. we treated the problem arising from the underregistration of births and indicated the needed adjustments. The estimate of underregistration at the national level has been done through backward projection of the census population under 10 years of age, and comparison with the births registered during the 10 years preceding the census. Since the censuses of 1900, 1911, and 1920 refer to December 1, the populations under 10 years of age of each census have been compared, respectively, with the births of 1891-1900, 1902-1911, and 1911-1920. Therefore, the estimated births are computed as follows:

$$Be = {}_5P_0 \times \frac{1_0}{{}_5L_0/5} + {}_5P_5 \times \frac{1_0}{{}_5L_5/5}$$

In 3.3. we explained that the computation of the coefficients for the backward projection has been based on the Princeton model life tables (South); the appropriate life tables have been selected through the combination of the rate of natural increase and of the death rate in the decades preceding the census, as indicated here below:

Period	*Death rate*	*Natural increase*
1891-1900	21.24	9.32
1902-1911	20.08	12.10
1911-1920	23.68[a]	8.77

In Table 46 we have reported the computations for the evaluation of underregistration. In 1891-1900, "registered" births are 4.1 percent below the "estimated" births; in the following decade (1902-1911) our computations show a slight excess (+0.2 percent) of registered over estimated births. This is probably the consequence of the "recuperation" of about 40,000 births in 1911, whose registration had been omitted in the preceding years. Omit-

[a] The very high value is imputable to the epidemic of influenza.

ting 40,000 births from the total births of 1902-1911, underregistration of the decade is about 2 percent.

It may be possible that the "revival" rate of 1.3057 adopted for the 1920 census population of 0-4 years old is too low. The mortality level of 1911-1920 was abnormally high because of the epidemic of influenza at the end of the decade. It is likely that the epidemic affected the very young age groups more than the older ones; therefore, the revival ratio should be increased accordingly. In this case, the difference of 17.8 percent between estimated and registered births should be proportionally reduced, which would reduce the overall (0-9) difference of 6.4 percent and come closer to the estimated difference for 1902-1911.

We must note also that in Portugal, as in Spain and in Italy, the census age distribution seems to be distorted in a particular way. The age group 0-4 is generally heavily undercounted, but part of the omitted units are recuperated in the following 5-9 age group, which generally appears to be overenumerated. This pattern is clearly demonstrated by the values of the differences between registered and estimated births reported in Table 46 (last column), bearing opposite signs for the age groups 0-4 and 5-9.

Given the lack of more detailed information about the level of underregistration in the various years, we have assumed that the births of 1888-1892 and 1900-1904 (employed for the computation of fertility measures) were equally underreported by 4.1 percent. This is for the whole country. For the various districts, the correction factors have been estimated as follows:

(1) In the first place, we have estimated the number of births with delayed registration in each district in 1911, subtracting from the births registered in 1911, the average number of births registered in 1908-1910 and 1912-1914.

(2) We have assumed that the number of births underreported in 1888-1892 and 1900-1904 (and equal, in relative terms and at the national level, to —4.1 percent) could be "allocated" between the districts proportionally to the number of births with delayed registration in 1911.

Table 46. Computations for the Evaluation of Underregistration

Age of census population	Census population	$\frac{l_0}{{}_5L_x/5}$	Estimated Births	Years of birth registration	Registered births	Registered / Estimated
			1891-1900			
0-4	637,009	1.2632	804,670	1896-1900	805,255	+ 0.1
5-9	623,524[a]	1.3871	864,890	1891-1895	795,773	− 6.0
Total	1,260,533		1,669,560		1,601,028	− 4.1
			1902-1911			
0-4	706,306	1.2478	881,329	1907-1911	943,391	+ 7.0
5-9	703,153	1.3606	956,710	1902-1906	898,559	− 6.1
Total	1,409,459		1,838,039		1,841,950	+ 0.2
			1911-1920			
0-4	604,132	1.3057	788,815	1916-1920	928,928	+17.8
5-9	683,886[b]	1.4632	1,000,662	1911-1915	975,480[c]	− 2.5
Total	1,288,018		1,789,477			+ 6.4

[a] For age 9 the census figure is 113,627, a value obviously underreported because of the age-heaping; the figure of 127,000 has been, therefore, substituted (127,000 is the average population in the ages of 9, 10, and 11 years).

[b] For age 9 same procedure as described in a; the adopted value is 131,295, instead of 128,610.

[c] From the 230,033 live births registered in 1911, we have subtracted 40,000 births that were registered in 1911 but probably took place in the preceding years.

(3) The number of registered births plus the number of births "allocated" as in (2) gives the total number of births adjusted for the computation of the fertility rates.

(4) The correction factors of each district (total number of adjusted births/total number of registered births) are reported below: 1.0: Porto; 1.01: Angra, Funchal, Castelo Branco; 1.02: Aveiro, Viana do Castelo, Horta, Ponta Delgada; 1.03: Guarda and Leiria; 1.04: Braga, Coimbra, Portalegre, Vila Real, Viseu; 1.06: Faro; 1.08: Beja, Lisbon, Bragança; 1.09: Évora.

Official Statistical Sources

Census Statistics

Estatística de Portugal, População, *Censo no 1° de janeiro 1864,* Lisbon, 1868.

Estatística de Portugal, População, *Censo no 1° de janeiro 1878,* Lisbon, 1881.

Direcção Geral de Estatística, *Censo da população do reino de Portugal no 1° de dezembro de 1890,* Vol. I, Lisbon, 1896; Vol. II, Lisbon, 1900.

Idem., Censo da população do reino de Portugal no 1° de dezembro de 1900, Resultados provisorios, Lisbon, 1901; Vol. I, Lisbon, 1905.

Idem., Censo da população de Portugal no 1° de dezembro de 1911, Part 1, Lisbon, 1913; Part 2 and 3, Lisbon, 1913; Part 4 and 5, Lisbon, 1914; Part 6, Lisbon, 1917.

Idem., Censo da população de Portugal no 1° de dezembro de 1920, Vol. I, Lisbon, 1923; Vol. II, Lisbon, 1925.

Idem., Censo da população de Portugal no 1° de dezembro de 1930, Vol. I, Lisbon, 1933; Vol. II, Lisbon, 1934; Vol. III, Lisbon, 1934; Vol. IV, Lisbon, 1934.

Instituto Nacional de Estatística, *Recenseamento geral da população no continente e ilhas adjacentes em 12 de dezembro de 1940,* Vol. I-XXV, Lisbon, 1945.

Idem., IX Recenseamento geral da população no continente e ilhas adjacentes em 15 de dezembro de 1950, Vol. I, II, and III, Lisbon, 1952-53.

Idem., X Recenseamento geral da população no continente e ilhas adjacentes (às 0 horas de 15 de dezembro de 1960), Vol. I-IV, Lisbon, 1964.

Direcção Geral de Estatística, *Censo extraordinario da população das cidades de Lisboa e Porto, 1° dezembro 1925,* Lisbon, 1927.

OFFICIAL STATISTICAL SOURCES

Vital Statistics

Direcção Geral do Commercio e Industria (then Direcção Geral de Estatística), *Movimento da população,* years 1887 (Lisbon, 1890), 1889-90, 1891-93, 1894-96, 1907-14, 1915-16, 1917-18 and 1920-21.

Arquivos do Instituto Central de Higiene (after Direcção Geral de Saûde) *Movimento fisiológico da população de Portugal,* 1913 (Lisbon, 1920), and every year until 1925.

Direcção Geral de Estatística, *Anuário demográfico,* yearbooks 1929-1967.

Other References

Aranha, et al., *Le Portugal,* Paris, no date.

Balbi, A., *Compendio di geografía,* Vol. I, Turin, 1840.

———. *Essai statistique sur le royaume de Portugal et d'Algarve, comparé aux autres états de l'Europe, et suivi d'un coup d'oeil sur l'état actuel des sciences, des lettres et des beaux arts parmi les Portugais des deux hémisphères,* Vol. I, Paris, 1822.

———. *Variétés politico-statistiques sur la monarchie Portugaise,* Paris, 1822.

Bettencourt, J. de Souza, "El fenomeno de la emigración Portuguesa," *Revista internacional de sociologia,* n. 68, 1959-60.

Birot, P., *Le Portugal. Etude de géographie régionale,* Paris, 1950.

Blanc, A., Drain, M., and Kayser, B., *L'Europe Méditerranéenne,* Paris, 1967.

Caldas, E. de Castro, and Loureiro, M. de Santos, *Regioes homogéneas no continente Português,* Lisbon, 1966.

Casa Nova, A., "Aspectos demográficos da população Portuguesa," *R.C.E.D.,* n. 10.

Coale, A. J., "Factors Associated with the Development of Low Fertility: an Historic Summary," *World Population Conference, 1965,* Vol. II.

Coale, A. J., and Demeny, P., *Regional Model Life Tables and Stable Populations,* Princeton, 1966.

da Costa, A. Rebelo, *Descripção topográfica e historica da cidade do Porto,* Porto, 1788.

de Barros, Soares, "Sobre a causa da diferente população em diversos tempos da Monarchia," *Memorias economicas da Academia Real das Sciências de Lisboa,* Vol. I, 1789.

Descamps, P. *Le Portugal,* Paris, 1935.

de Vasconcellos, J. Leite, *Etnografia Portuguesa,* Lisbon, Vol. III, 1942, Vol. IV, 1958.

Dias, J., "Minho, Tras-os-Montes, Haut Douro," *Congrès international de géographie,* Lisbon, 1949.

Feio, M., "Le bas Alentejo et l'Algarve," *Congrès international de géographie,* Lisbon, 1949.

Ferro, G., “Per uno studio delle città Portoghesi,” *Annali di ricerche e studi di geografia,* Vol. XIV.

———. “Le frontiere del Portogallo e la sua suddivisione regionale,” *Rivista geografica Italiana,* Vol. LXXI, 1964.

Garrett, A. Almeida, “Os problemas da natalidade,” *R.C.E.D.*, n. 2, 3, 5.

Girão, A. de Amorim, *Geografía de Portugal,* Porto, 1941.

———. “Origens e evolução do urbanismo em Portugal,” *R.C.E.D.*, n. 1, 1945.

Hajnal, J., "European Marriage Patterns in Perspective,” in *Population in History,* edited by D. V. Glass and D. E. C. Eversley, London, 1965.

Jorge, R., *Demographia e hygiene da cidade do Porto,* Porto, 1899.

Livi Bacci, M., “Il declino della fecondita della popolazione Italiana nell' ultimo secolo,” *Statistica,* Vol. XXV, 1965.

———. “Sur les régions de l'Europe où la fécondité demeure élevée,” *European Population Conference, Strasbourg, 1966,* Vol. I.

———. “Fertility and Nuptiality Changes in Spain from the Late 18th to the Early 20th Century,” Part 2, *Population Studies,* Vol. XXIII, 1967.

Machado, J. T. Montalvão, “Alguns aspectos da natalidade,” *R.C.E.D.*, n. 10.

———. “No centenario do I censo populacional Português,” *R.C.E.D.*, n. 16, 1965.

Moraes, J. J. Paes, “Tábuas de extinção de solteiros para 1940 e 1950,” *R.C.E.D.*, n. 9.

———. “Alguns aspectos demograficos da população Portuguesa,” *Estudos, Instituto Nacional de Estatística,* n. 18, Lisbon, 1960.

Organization for Economic Cooperation and Development, “Le Portugal,” in *Etudes économiques de l'O.C.D.E.*, Paris, 1964.

Pery, G., *Statistique du Portugal et des colonies,* Lisbon, 1878.

Portugal, Instituto Nacional de Estatística, *Subsídios para a história da estatística em Portugal,* Vol. II, *Taboas topograficas e estatísticas, 1801,* Lisbon, 1948.

Ribeiro, O., "Portugal," in *Geografía de España y Portugal*, edited by M. de Teran, Vol. v, Barcelona, 1955.

Sampaio, A., *Estudos históricos e económicos*, Vol. I, Porto, 1923.

Silbert, A., *Le Portugal Méditerranéen*, Vol. I, Paris, 1966.

United Nations, *Demographic Yearbook, 1965*, New York, 1966.

Valenti, J. Vilá, *La Péninsule Ibérique*, Paris, 1968.

Villier, F., *Portogallo*, Milan, 1961.

Whelpton, P. K., Campbell, A. A., and Patterson, J. E., *Fertility and Family Planning in the United States*, Princeton, 1966.

Index

INDEX

GPSR Authorized Representative: Easy Access System Europe - Mustamäe tee 50, 10621 Tallinn, Estonia, gpsr.requests@easproject.com

www.ingramcontent.com/pod-product-compliance
Ingram Content Group UK Ltd.
Pitfield, Milton Keynes, MK11 3LW, UK
UKHW021457290926
475585UK00012B/19